Everyday Audiology

A Practical Guide for Health Care Professionals

Audiology Editor-in-Chief
Brad A. Stach, Ph.D.

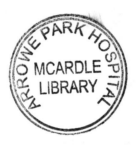

Everyday Audiology

A Practical Guide for Health Care Professionals

Kazunari J. Koike, Ph.D.

Department of Otolaryngology–Head and Neck Surgery
West Virginia University Health Sciences Center
Morgantown, West Virginia

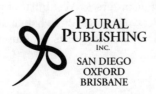

PLURAL
PUBLISHING
INC.

SAN DIEGO
OXFORD
BRISBANE

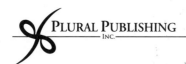

5521 Ruffin Road
San Diego, CA 92123

e-mail: info@pluralpublishing.com
Web site: http://www.pluralpublishing.com

49 Bath Street
Abingdon, Oxfordshire OX14 1EA
United Kingdom

Typeset in 11/13 Garamond by Flanagan's Publishing Services, Inc.
Printed in the United States of America by McNaughton and Gunn.

Library of Congress Cataloging-in-Publication Data

Koike, Kazunari J.
   Everyday audiology : a practical guide for health care professionals / Kazunari J.
Koike.
      p. ; cm.
   Includes bibliographical references and index.
   ISBN-13: 978-1-59756-088-7 (softcover)
   ISBN-10: 1-59756-088-X (softcover)
   1. Audiology. 2. Hearing disorders 3. Vestibular apparatus–Diseases.
[DNLM: 1. Hearing Disorders–diagnosis. 2. Rehabilitation of Hearing Impaired. 3.
Dizziness. 4. Hearing Aids. 5. Hearing Tests. 6. Musculoskeletal Equilibrium.
WV 270 K79e 2006] I. Title.
RF290.K64 2006
617.8–dc22

                                                                      2006005774

Contents

Foreword

Kaz Koike has developed an excellent guide to help not just otolaryngology residents but also practitioners to understand the many audiologic and vestibular tests that we frequently use to help diagnose and treat our patients. Dr. Koike has a gift for explaining complicated tests in a concise and simple fashion. This monograph is a valuable tool for all who are interested in the field of audiology and in vestibular testing.

Stephen J. Wetmore, M.D., M.B.A.
Professor and Chair
Department of Otolaryngology
West Virginia University School of Medicine

Preface

This textbook was originally written primarily for ENT residents. Its focus is to help residents understand the essentials of audiology in a very compressed period of time without sacrificing accuracy. I assume that each resident will continue to seek further knowledge from other resources as this textbook is not designed to provide exhaustive details of various audiologic techniques. I encourage residents to ask "nearby audiologists" any questions regarding the audiologic examination of patients, because only through knowledge of that process can audiology become practical and clinically relevant.

This textbook is also a culmination of case reports conducted by our clinical audiologists, Mary Archer, Susan Cappellini, Holly Hurley, Liesl Perry, and Leslie Purcell and much feedback from our ENT residents, current and past. I remain thankful for having such support. I would also like to acknowledge Dr. Stephen Wetmore, Chair of the Department, for his continuous encouragement to complete this textbook for our residents.

I have come to the conclusion that this book can be useful not only to ENT residents but also to other health care professionals including otolaryngologists, family medicine physicians, pediatricians, medical students, audiologists, audiology students, teachers of the hearing impaired, hearing instrument specialists, speech-language pathologists who work with hearing-impaired children, and even physical therapists who provide rehabilitation to patients with balance disorders.

Audiology is my lifelong profession, and I practice it in the clinic every day, hopefully to have a positive impact on the lives of people with hearing or balance disorders. If you are a chef, you cook every day. If you are a car mechanic, you work on cars every day. So, I decided to title my book, "Everyday Audiology."

KJK

Overview

Hearing loss, both acute and chronic, is a common complaint seen among patients of all ages. This textbook is an attempt to visually depict audiologic diagnostic procedures, including the history and physical examination of hearing. It further describes appropriate use and interpretation of audiologic evaluations. It is essential that physicians understand what kind of audiologic evaluations are available, when they are useful, and how to interpret the results meaningfully for proper diagnosis and treatment of hearing problems.

The textbook is divided into three parts: Part I, Evaluation of Hearing Disorders; Part II, Evaluation of Balance Disorders; and Part III, Rehabilitation of Hearing Disorders. Frequently used audiology terminology and significant clinical criteria are printed in bold. The Current Procedural Terminology (CPT) code, if available, is listed under each test procedure.

PART I

Evaluation of Hearing Disorders

After taking a thorough case history from the patient, physicians must determine the possible site of hearing loss, if any. The most common sites of hearing loss, whether acute or chronic, are either the middle ear or the inner ear (Fig. 1). Although many technical aspects of the audiologic evaluation are beyond the scope of this textbook, a close working relationship between physician and audiologist, as well as a basic understanding of what each evaluation offers, are essential for a proper diagnosis of hearing loss.

A synopsis of how various audiologic evaluations are used for differential diagnosis is summarized in Table 1.

Table 1. Summary of Audiologic Evaluations for Differential Diagnosis.

Outer & Middle Ears	Inner Ear	Retrocochlear
Audiogram	Audiogram	Audiogram
Tympanogram	Acoustic Reflex	AR Decay
	Threshold ABR	Neurologic ABR
	ASSR	CAP
	ECoG	
	OAE	
	ENG/VNG	

Note: ABR = auditory brainstem response; AR = acoustic reflex; ASSR = auditory steady state response; CAP = central auditory processing; ECoG = electrocochleography; ENG = electronystagmography; OAE = otoacoustic emissions; VNG = videonystagmography.

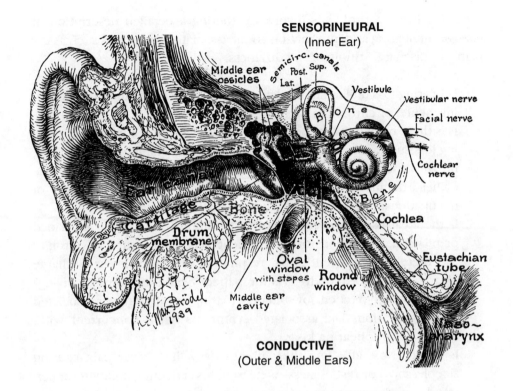

Figure 1. A classic drawing of the human ear by Brodel (1946). A coronal view of the outer ear, middle ear, and inner ear depicts conductive (outer and middle ears) and sensorineural (inner ear) mechanisms of the human ear. (From Brodel, M. [1946] *Three unpublished drawings of the anatomy of the human ear.* Philadelphia, PA: W.B. Saunders. Copyright 1946 by W.B. Saunders. Reprinted with permission.)

History

Assessing hearing problems involves gathering a detailed description of changes in hearing and information about associated symptoms such as ear pain, ear discharge, tinnitus, and dizziness.

1. Is hearing loss unilateral or bilateral, continuous, intermittent, fluctuating, acute, or chronic in nature?
2. Has there been a recent or past illness or event that could cause hearing loss such as sudden exposure to loud noise, viral illness, meningitis, measles, mumps, syphilis, high fever, diuretic use, aminoglycoside use, or head trauma? Is there any family history of hearing loss, history of occupational noise exposure, ear surgery, or hearing aid use?
3. Is there ear pain, discharge, tinnitus, or dizziness? Are these one-sided or bilateral, continuous or intermittent, recurrent, acute, or chronic? Has there been a recent upper respiratory infection? Is ear discharge clear, purulent, or bloody? Has the patient been swimming or diving? Is tinnitus high-pitched, low-pitched, roaring or pulsating, or associated with medication? Did associated symptoms begin concurrent with, before, or after hearing loss?
4. Is hearing loss affecting the patient's daily life? Is ear pain causing sleeplessness or restlessness? Is hearing loss affecting ability to understand speech or even to pronounce speech sounds correctly?

Various questionnaires have been developed to examine the effects of hearing loss on a patient's social and emotional adjustment (Koike, Hurst, & Wetmore, 1994; Ventry & Weinstein, 1982). The Hearing Handicap Inventory for the Elderly-Screening (HHIE-S) can be used as such a "self-assessment" tool (Fig. 2). It has been found to be a reliable measure and is closely correlated to standard audiometric data (Ventry & Weinstein, 1983; Weinstein & Ventry, 1983).

Hearing Handicap Inventory for the Elderly
Screening Version (HHIE-S)

Please answer "yes" or "no" to "sometimes" to each of the following items. Do not skip a question if you avoid a situation because of a hearing problem. If you use a hearing aid, please answer the way you hear without the aid.

		Yes (4)	Some-times (2)	No (0)
E-1	Does a hearing problem cause you to feel embarrassed when meeting new people?			
E-2	Does a hearing problem cause you to feel frustrated when talking to members of your family?			
S-1	Do you have difficulty hearing when someone speaks in a whisper?			
E-3	Do you feel handicapped by a hearing problem?			
S-2	Does a hearing problem cause you difficulty when visiting friends, relatives, or neighbors?			
S-3	Does a hearing problem cause you to attend religious services less often than you would like?			
E-4	Does a hearing problem cause you to have arguments with family members?			
S-4	Does a hearing problem cause you difficulty when listening to TV or radio?			
E-5	Do you feel that any difficulty with your hearing limits or hampers your personal or social life?			
S-5	Does a hearing problem cause you difficulty when in a restaurant with relatives or friends?			

Handicap Score: Yes (4) x _____ + Sometimes (2) x _____ + No (0) x _____ = _____

Handicap Score	*Degree of Handicap*	*Probability of Hearing Loss*
0-10	No handicap/No referral	13%
12-24	Mild-Moderate Handicap	50%
26-40	Severe Handicap	84%

Figure 2. A questionnaire form for the HHIE-S (adapted from Ventry & Weinstein, 1983). Patients can fill out the form while they wait for formal audiometric testing. It may be combined with an audiogram as a counseling tool. (Adapted with permission from Ventry, I. M., & Weinstein, B. M. [1983], Identification of elderly people with hearing problems. *Asha, 25*, 37–42. Copyright 1983 American Speech and Hearing Association.)

Audiogram

(CPT Codes: 92557, 92552, 92553)

An audiogram is a graph of hearing (Fig. 3). It depicts the degree and type of hearing loss at designated frequencies. It can be performed whenever there is a question of hearing loss based on the patient's complaints of acute ear infections, chronic ear disease, gradual hearing decline over the years, sudden hearing loss, hereditary or progressive hearing loss, and/or the complaint of dizziness or tinnitus.

The audiometric evaluation can be performed for patients of all ages, although specific techniques vary according to the patient's age and cognitive level.

Hearing Level

Hearing level (HL) is determined by asking the patient to respond (e.g., raise the hand, push the button) to stimuli, typically pure tones of different frequencies. HL is the **threshold** (minimal level) where a response is obtained **50% of the time** (e.g., 2 out of 4 trials) at a particular frequency. It is determined by a **bracketing** technique, where the stimulus level is raised in a 5-dB increment as long as the patient does not respond to the stimulus while the presentation level is lowered in a 10-dB increment when there is a positive response.

Calibration and Equal-Loudness Contours

The sensitivity of the human ear is unequal across different frequencies unlike the straight line depicted in the audiogram. The curves that depict equal loudness of various pure tones, compared to the loudness of a 1000-Hz tone by normal hearing listeners are called "**equal-loudness contours**" (Robinson & Dadson, 1956; see reference note). Therefore, in the "standard" audiogram, the **Minimum Audible Field (MAF)** measured in **dB sound pressure level (SPL)** is converted (or **calibrated**) to 0 dB HL according to the American National Standard Institute (ANSI, 1969; see reference note).

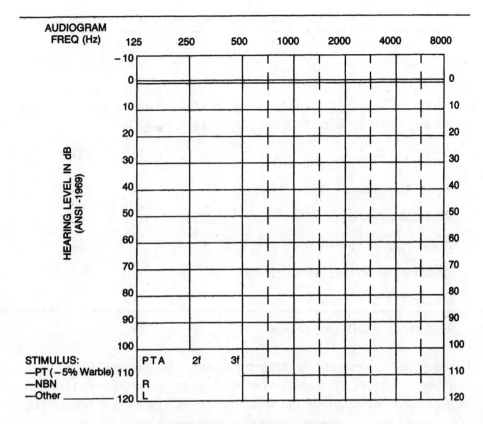

Figure 3. Standard audiogram with 0 dB HL being calibrated according to ANSI-1969. Audimetric symbols (ASHA, 1990) below indicate air conduction, bone conduction thresholds for the right and left ear, and sound field thresholds. Symbols for unmasked and masked conditions are also shown.

Degree of Hearing Loss

The degree of hearing loss can be categorized as follows (recommended by Goodman, 1965; modified by Clark, 1981) (Figs. 4 and 5):

Normal: −10 to 15 dB;

Slight/Borderline: 16 to 25 dB;

Mild: 26 to 40 dB;

Moderate: 41 to 55 dB;

Moderately severe: 56 to 70 dB;

Severe: 71 to 90 dB;

Profound: 91 dB or greater.

It is useful to understand how different degrees of hearing loss affect human communication as clinicians try to explain the impact of hearing problems to patients or their parents and family members. The level of normal conversational speech averages around 50 dB, ranging from 20 dB for whispered speech to 65 dB for loud talking voices (see lighter shading area in Figs. 4 and 5). Amplification is recommended for hearing losses exceeding the mild degree, and the need for rehabilitation becomes more obligatory as the degree worsens. Again, a questionnaire like the HHIE-S could delineate how much the patient is subjectively perceiving communication difficulty and could be used as a counseling tool. Furthermore, clinicians should be aware that in children even a minimal amount of hearing loss, especially if prolonged, can affect learning and proper development of speech and language (Bess, 1985; Tharpe & Bess, 1999). The effects become more significant as the degree of the hearing loss increases.

The Effects of Hearing Loss on Human Communication

Slight to Mild

Hears well in a quiet room while listening to one or two people

Difficulty understanding only in selected conditions such as listening in noise or understanding softly spoken speech

Possible need for amplification

Concern for speech and language development; academic concern

Moderate

Begins to have difficulty understanding even in ideal conditions

Requires people to talk louder even at closer distances (e.g., within 3 to 5 feet)

Increased need for amplification

Increased need for visual cues such as lip-reading

Definite concern for speech and language development

Severe

Needs others to begin to alter the normal mode of speech communication

Needs to speak to them with a loud voice even within one foot

Affects speech production and will require speech therapy

Cannot communicate without amplification.

Profound

Amplification alone may not be sufficient means of communication

May need a means of communication other than the auditory mode

Total communication, manual signs, and/or cochlear implantation may be indicated

Type of Hearing Loss

The type of hearing loss is determined by comparing the test results from two types of measurements: an **air-conduction (AC) test** and a **bone-conduction (BC) test**. The AC test literally means that the testing is done by presenting the stimulus through earphones, thus transmitting the sound to the inner ear through the air. In this method, the sounds must go through the ear canal, middle ear cavity, and then to the cochlea where the sensory receptors (i.e., hair cells) of hearing are located. In the BC test, the sounds are transmitted to the inner ear directly through vibration of the temporal bone, thus bypassing the outer and middle ear structures (like the tuning fork placement on the mastoid during the Rinne test).

Sensorineural Hearing Loss

A **sensorineural hearing loss (SNHL)** is a hearing loss primarily due to inner ear (sensory hair cells) and/or VIIIth nerve (neural) pathology (Fig. 4). The audiogram depicts the AC thresholds overlapping with the BC thresholds (equivalent to a positive Rinne). No additional loss is expected from outer and middle ear pathology. SNHL with acute onset is relatively rare, but the etiologies could include autoimmune disease, idiopathic sudden hearing loss, trauma, and ototoxicity. Most SNHL is permanent with common etiologies including aging (i.e., **presbycusis**) (Maurer & Rupp, 1979, see reference note), noise (i.e., **noise-induced hearing loss, NIHL**) (Melnick, 1978, see reference note; Miller, 1986), ototoxicity (Roland & Rutka, 2004), inner ear diseases (e.g., Ménière's disease), retrocochlear pathology (e.g., acoustic neuroma), and hereditary hearing loss. SNHL beyond a mild degree typically requires some rehabilitation such as hearing aids, assistive listening devices, and aural rehabilitation.

SENSORINEURAL HEARING LOSS
(SNHL)

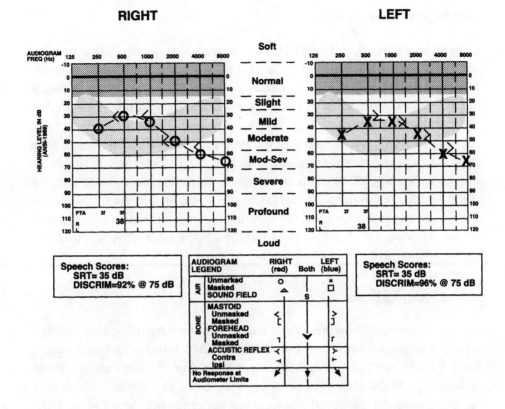

Figure 4. Audiogram of a bilateral mild-to-moderately severe SNHL. Circles (often in red) = right AC thresholds; crosses (often in blue) = left AC thresholds; right open brackets = right BC thresholds; left open brackets = left BC thresholds. Normal hearing is shown by the shading, while the range of normal speech conversation is shown by lighter shading.

Conductive Hearing Loss

A **conductive hearing loss (CHL)** is a hearing loss primarily due to outer and middle ear pathologies (Fig. 5). The BC thresholds are better than the AC thresholds (equivalent to a negative Rinne). This difference between the AC and BC thresholds is called an **air-bone gap**, and is attributed to outer and middle ear pathology "blocking" sound transmission. Most CHL, contrary to SNHL, is temporary. Common etiologies include swimmer's ear, otitis media, TM perforation, cholesteatoma, and otosclerosis. It should be emphasized that CHL is often reversible with appropriate treatment that could include spontaneous recovery, medication, and/or surgery. Chronic CHL could result from recurrent otitis media, TM perforation, chronic middle ear diseases, and deformities of the ear associated with syndromes that commonly involve the head and neck.

Mixed Hearing Loss

A third category of hearing loss is called a **mixed hearing loss (MHL)**, which is simply a combination of SNHL and CHL. It occurs when a patient has an SNHL with depressed BC thresholds, but also has an additional conductive component depicted by the air-bone gap across frequencies. MHL is commonly observed among adult patients with pre-existing SNHL (e.g., presbycusis, NIHL) in addition to common middle ear pathologies (e.g., middle ear effusion, TM perforation, cholesteatoma).

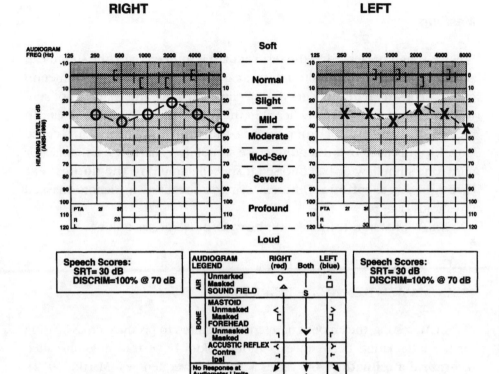

Figure 5. Audiogram of a bilateral mild CHL. Square open brackets indicate the "masked" BC thresholds when masking noise is used to eliminate the non-test ear from responding. Effective masking (EM) of about 60 dB (70 dB–40 dB IA plus CHL of 30 dB) also needs to be presented to the contralateral nontest ear during speech discrimination presented at 70 dB for the test ear.

Masking

When a sound presented to the test ear (TE) is loud enough, the sound can also be heard in the opposite nontest ear (NTE). When this phenomenon called "**cross-hearing**" occurs during clinical testing, the tester is not sure whether the stimulus is truly heard in the test ear or in the nontest ear. To prevent the nontest ear from hearing the stimulus, a technique called "**masking**" is used by presenting noise stimuli (e.g. narrow-band noise for pure tone stimuli, wide-band noise for speech stimuli) **to the nontest ear through the earphone**. Different symbols are used to denote masked thresholds (Fig. 5).

Rules for **when to mask** and **how to mask** are as follows.

AC: **MASK WHEN $AC_{TE} - BC_{NTE} \geq 40$ dB**

BC: **MASK WHEN $AC_{TE} - BC_{TE} \geq 10$ dB**

In AC testing, the amount of intensity required to produce cross-hearing (or the attenuation between ears though skull bone transmission called **interaural attenuation, IA**) varies across the frequencies (Martin, 1972). For example, the range of IA for the 250 Hz tone is from 50 to 80 dB while the range for the 2000 Hz tone is 45 to 75 dB. Traditionally, **IA of 40 dB** is used for all pure tone frequencies as a conservative value when we determine the need for masking. This rule of thumb can also apply to speech stimuli (see Fig. 5).

In BC testing, cross-hearing to the nontest ear occurs almost every time the signal is presented to the test ear as the **IA for BC is nearly 0 dB**. Do we always need to mask during the BC testing? In fact, some audiologists always do. A practical compromise that most audiologists have adopted, however, is to mask when a significant air-bone gap (10 dB or greater) is observed in the test ear. Then, masking should be used in **the nontest ear through the earphone** to ensure that the patient is responding to the stimuli being heard in the test ear, not in the nontest ear.

Effective Masking

If the **effective masking level** of the audiometer is calibrated, the amount of masking noise needed to eliminate the sensation of the pure tone stimulus is the same as the pure tone level (i.e., 10 dB masking noise is needed to mask 10 dB pure tone signal). A safeguard of an additional 10 dB is traditionally added; thus the amount of initial masking noise is usually set to **10 dB above the AC threshold of the nontest ear**. When this initial level of masking is presented to the nontest ear and the stimulus to the test ear can still be heard in the test ear, the **minimum effective masking (EM)** is established and you can take the original threshold as a true threshold. However, if the sensation of the stimulus at the initial threshold disappears with masking, you assume that the original stimulus must have been heard from the nontest ear due to cross-hearing, thus the level of the pure tone stimulus must be raised, typically in 5-dB increments. If the stimulus is heard again, the masking level must also be raised another 5 dB. This process is called the "**plateau**" technique (Hood, 1960). At least a 15-dB plateau needs to be established to determine the "true" threshold. That is, the sensation of the stimulus must be maintained in the test ear, while the masking level is raised at least 15 to 20 dB in the nontest ear.

For patients with mild-to-moderate bilateral CHL, a phenomenon called **overmasking** may occur. For example, due to the need to provide masking through earphones to the nontest ear with 40 dB HL or even greater, the level of masking noise begins to cross over back to the test ear, thus creating a "masking dilemma." Insert probe earphones that have greater IA values may provide an alternative way to overcome this dilemma (Black, Oyer, & Seyfried, 1991; Clemis, Ballard, & Killion, 1986).

Speech Reception Threshold and Discrimination

(CPT Code: 92556)

Although the audiogram (Figs. 4 and 5, see speech scores) uses a tone to elicit a response from the patient, the **speech reception threshold (SRT)** indicates how soft the patient can understand speech using spondee words with equal stress for each syllable such as "hotdog" and "baseball," commonly known as **CID W-1** words, developed at the Central Institute for the Deaf (Hirsh et al., 1952; Hudgins et al., 1947).

The SRT and the **pure tone average (PTA)** at 500, 1000, and 2000 Hz (or two best frequencies) should agree within 10 dB in order for an audiogram to have good reliability. A significant deviation from this pattern (e.g., SRT significantly better than the PTA) should be interpreted with caution for suspicion of nonorganic hearing loss.

Speech discrimination scores show how well the patient understands speech that is presented at a comfortable listening level (Figs. 4 and 5, see speech scores). For example, patients with CHL typically produce good discrimination scores once speech is presented at reasonable **loudness**. However, some individuals with SNHL have lost not only the ability to detect sound (loudness), but also the ability to **discriminate** words like "six" versus "fix." They complain, "I can *hear* you talking, but don't *understand* it." Furthermore, patients with "disproportionately poor" speech discrimination scores (Yellin, Jerger, & Fifer, 1989; see reference note) need to be carefully screened for Ménière's disease, acoustic neuroma, or even nonorganic hearing loss.

The **phonetically balanced (PB)** lists of monosyllabic words, such as the **CID W-22** (Hirsh et al., 1952; Hudgins et al., 1947), **PB-K** (Kindergarten, used for children; Haskins, 1949), or the **NU 6** (developed at Northwestern University) are balanced in terms of phoneme frequency of occurrence in conversational speech and have been commonly used in audiology practice. It was assumed that all speech sounds must be included to test hearing (Hudgins et al., 1947) and phonetic balancing ensured homogeneity across different lists (Hirsh et al., 1952). Other more recently developed word lists, based on different linguistic theories, have been used for different applications, such as hearing aid or cochlear implant evaluations. For example, **Lexical Neighborhood Test (LNT)** and **Multisyllabic LNT (MLNT)** comprise word lists based on both word frequency and lexical similarity (or "neighborhoods") (Kirk, Pisoni, & Osberger, 1995). The word "old" is considered an "easy" word because it occurs with high frequency in sparse phoneme neighborhoods. The word "bed" is a "hard" word because it occurs less frequently but in dense phoneme neighborhoods, slightly differing from words like bet, red, fed, bad, and so forth by only one phoneme substitution. Research seems to indicate that listeners are sensitive to the composition of these lists and typically produce better scores when they are compared with traditional PB lists. Another commonly used test, **Hearing in Noise Test (HINT)** consists of sentences with a background noise for the purpose of examining speech understanding in noisy conditions because hearing-impaired listeners have more difficulty understanding in noise (Nilson, Soli, & Sullivan, 1994)

Examples of the CID W-1 Spondee Words

greyhound, schoolboy, inkwell, whitewash, pancake, hotdog, baseball, birthday, toothbrush, playground, sidewalk

Examples of the CID W-22 Words

mew, bathe, felt, ache, knees, twins, thing, stove, true, skin

(These 10 words are also ordered according to the degree of difficulty, and often referred to as **Mayo 10** bearing the name of the Mayo Clinic that developed it.)

Examples of the CID PB-K Words

please, great, sled, pants, rat, bad, pinch, such, bus, need

Examples of the HINT Sentences

(A/The) boy fell from (a/the) window.

(A/The) wife helped her husband.

Big dogs can be dangerous.

Tuning Fork Testing

Although the audiogram provides both qualitative and quantitative information with regard to hearing loss, further distinguishing of conductive from sensorineural hearing loss "qualitatively" can be performed with tuning fork testing as part of an ENT physical examination. Commonly performed tests are the Rinne and Weber tests.

The **Rinne** test is most sensitive using a 256-Hz fork but a 512-Hz fork can be used and is acceptable. The base of the lightly vibrating tuning fork is placed on the mastoid bone, level with the ear canal (Fig. 6A) and compared to loudness level when the tines of the tuning fork are held near the ear canal (Fig. 6B). With normal hearing and sensorineural loss the sound is audibly louder through air than through bone. This is called a *positive* **Rinne**. With conductive loss it is heard louder through bone than air. This is a *negative* **Rinne**. Usually conductive loss of more than 25 dB is required to make BC better than AC. This phenomenon is often referred to as a "**converted fork**." In addition to formal audiometric information, some physicians use an observation of converted forks at more than two frequencies during a physical exam as an indication for surgical intervention of otosclerosis.

The **Weber** test (Fig. 6C) is performed with a 512 Hz fork that is struck until lightly vibrating and then is placed on the center of the forehead. A normal result (or ears with symmetric hearing loss) is sound heard as equally loud in both ears. Thus, there is no **lateralization** of sound. In conductive loss, sound is louder in the impaired ear (poorer ear) whereas in sensorineural loss the sound is louder in the unaffected ear (or better ear), provided asymmetry exists. To distinguish between "conductive" and "sensorineural," the Weber test results must be interpreted in combination with the Rinne test.

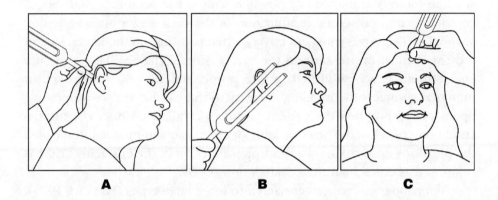

Figure 6. Different tuning fork placements for Rinne (*A and B*) and Weber (*C*) Tests

Tympanogram

(CPT Code: 92567)

A tympanogram depicts how well the tympanic membrane (TM) moves at varying air pressure points in the ear canal (Fig. 7). It can be performed anytime there is a question of possible middle ear pathology and should complement an otoscopic examination of the ear using a pneumatic otoscope. The TM moves most effectively when pressure on the lateral side of the TM is equal to pressure on the medial side of the TM. This "pressure equalization" is accomplished by the proper function of the eustachian tube that connects the middle ear cavity to the nasal cavity, as it normally opens or closes when the patient yawns or swallows. Under the normal condition, it is closed. The constantly open eustachian tube is often called the **patulous** eustachian tube. Improper function of the eustachian tube is diagnosed as eustachian tube dysfunction (ETD).

Tympanograms are categorized into three main types (Harford, 1975). In **Type A**, the tympanometric peaks fall within the normal range (the shaded area). In **Type B**, no distinct peak is observed, indicating low TM mobility. Always check the measurement of the ear canal volume (technically referred to as **physical volume**). The ear canal volume can be measured with the TM in a position of poor compliance, clamped at +200 mm/H_2O (daPa) air pressure, sometimes called "**Positive Pressure Test**," and may be performed as part of **Static Compliance Test** (Northern, 1975; see reference note). A normal ear canal volume (NV) should be between 0.3 and 1.0 for children and 0.5 to 2.0 for adults, and should **not exceed 1.0 cc for the average child** and **2.0 cc for the average adult**. If a large volume (LV) (e.g., often exceeding 4.0 or 5.0) is observed, Type B_{LV} indicates an open ventilation tube or a perforation. ***This must be verified by otoscopy***. In **Type C**, the peak falls in the negative pressure range beyond −100 daPa, indicating some degree of ETD. Variations of TM mobility (e.g., Type A_D, deep; Type A_S, shallow) can be associated with possible middle ear pathologies (e.g., ossicular discontinuity, otosclerosis), and need to be correlated with otoscopy.

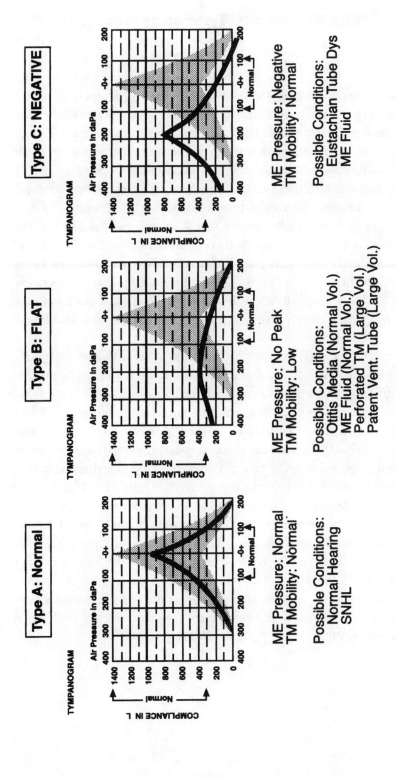

Figure 7. Tympanograms and possible conditions associated with each tympanogram. The vertical axis indicates the TM mobility (technically called "compliance"), while the horizontal axis indicates the middle ear (ME) pressure ranging from +200 mmH$_2$O (daPa in new standard) to 0 atmospheric pressure and further down to –400 daPa.

21

High-Frequency Tympanogram

(CPT Code: 92567)

A conventional tympanometer is accompanied by a probe assembly which consists of a microphone, a receiver, and a manometer to artificially alter air pressure inside the ear canal. The microphone is to detect any change in sound pressure level (SPL) inside the sealed ear canal cavity; hence, the only actual measurements during all the tympanometric tests are done in terms of SPL, then converted to various measures (e.g., compliance, volume). The receiver (equivalent to a miniature loudspeaker) is designed to constantly emit a probe tone with the frequency typically set to 226 Hz. The tympanogram described in the previous section uses this "low-frequency" probe tone to primarily measure the "stiffness" of the tympanic membrane (TM), of which the effect is most significant in the low frequencies. Remember, "Stiffness attenuates low frequencies." A typical clinical example is a low-frequency conductive hearing loss associated with middle ear effusion that "stiffens" the TM mobility.

However, the validity of this conventional tympanogram for young infants has been questioned through recent studies which indicate that "normal" tympanograms could erroneously reflect the mobility of soft tissue inside the ear canal, especially in young infants before 6 months of age, instead of truly measuring the mobility of the TM (Kei et al., 2003; McKinley, Grose, & Roush, 1997). Thus, a normal-appearing tympanogram can be obtained among infants who, in fact, may have reduced eardrum mobility. To overcome this dilemma, tympanometry using a high-frequency probe tone such as 1000 Hz has been introduced as an alternative with the notion that a relatively higher frequency probe may not be influenced by the flaccid soft tissue of the infant ear canal, but at the same time measuring the mobility of the eardrum (Fig. 8). Studies that utilized the high-frequency tympanogram (i.e., 1000-Hz probe tone) yielded a passing result in over 90% of normal neonate ears that also produced normal OAE results with the assumption that normal OAE results must presume normal middle ear function (Kei et al., 2003; Margolis et al., 2003).

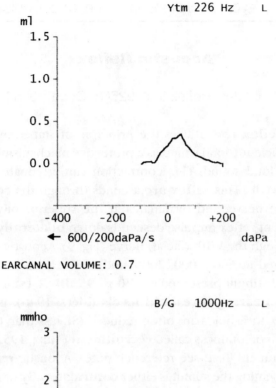

Ytm 226 Hz   L

ml
1.5
1.0
0.5
0.0

-400   -200   0   +200
◄ 600/200daPa/s   daPa

EARCANAL VOLUME: 0.7

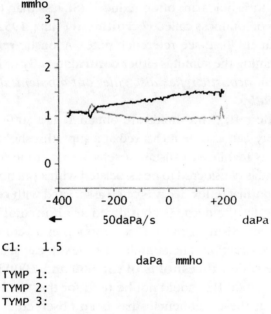

B/G 1000Hz   L

mmho
3
2
1
0

-400   -200   0   +200
◄ 50daPa/s   daPa

C1:   1.5

daPa mmho
TYMP 1:
TYMP 2:
TYMP 3:

Figure 8. Normal tympanogram using a 226-Hz probe tone (*top*), yet the tympanogram using a 1000 Hz probe tone (*bottom*) resulted in a flat Type B pattern, more accurately reflecting reduced eardrum mobility from a 7-week infant with suspicion of middle ear effusion.

Acoustic Reflex

(CPT Codes: Reflex test, 92568; Decay, 92569)

The **acoustic reflex test** utilizes the principle of stapedius muscle contraction to a sufficiently loud sound as a protective mechanism of the human ear against the loud sound. This contraction can attenuate an incoming sound by 5 to 10 dB. This **reflex arc** ascends through the cochlea via the VIIIth (auditory) nerve, and terminates at the superior olivary complex where the efferent reflex impulse descends down **bilaterally** to the stapedial muscle through the VIIth (facial) nerve (Fig. 9). Acoustic reflex thresholds are measured at 500, 1000, 2000, and 4000 Hz and can be elicited when the sound stimuli presented are **70 to 95 dB SL (sensation level) above normal hearing threshold levels** (Metz, 1946). In the sensorineural ear, reflex thresholds are often reduced (SL less than 60 dB) due to abnormal growth of loudness called **recruitment** (Metz, 1952; often called the Metz Recruitment Test; see reference note). Acoustic reflexes can be obtained by presenting the stimulus either **contralaterally** or **ipsilaterally**. *The presence of an acoustic reflex also rules out a potential diagnosis of auditory neuropathy.*

Once acoustic reflex thresholds are obtained at a sufficient stimulus level, **reflex decay** can also be measured at a suprathreshold level. Reflex decay is defined as inability to sustain a sensation of tone for a specified amount of time and is considered to be associated with a phenomenon called "**adaptation.**" Abnormal reflex decay is often associated with **retrocochlear pathology**. Typically, the decay is considered as **abnormal if there is a 50% or more reduction** in the reflex contraction as compared to the original level of contraction. The stimuli for reflex decay are presented **at 10 dB above the reflex thresholds of the 500 and 1000 Hz tone**. The frequencies above 2000 Hz should not be used for this test because some significant decay at these frequencies has been observed even in normal ears (Givens & Seidemann, 1979; Jerger, Jerger, & Mauldin, 1972).

CONTRALATERAL ACOUSTIC REFLEX

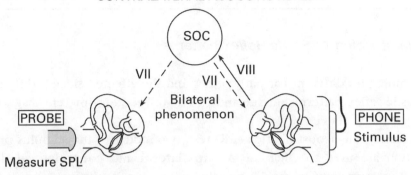

Is there stapedial m. contraction
as a result of the *contralateral*
sound stimulation?

Is the stimulus loud enough?

IPSILATERAL ACOUSTIC REFLEX

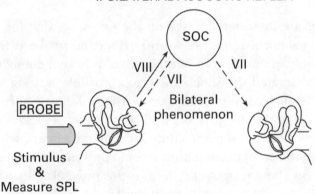

Is the stimulus loud enough?

Is there stapedial m. contraction
as a result of the *ipsilateral*
sound stimulation?

Figure 9. Contralateral and ipsilateral acoustic reflex arc.

Understanding Acoustic Reflex Patterns

Depending on different ear pathologies and the affected side(s), different acoustic reflex patterns emerge and can be utilized for different diagnosis (Jerger, 1975) (Table 2).

During the acoustic reflex (AR) test, two modes of the stimulus presentation are used to elicit the AR: **ipsilateral** and **contralateral**. The actual measurement of the AR muscle contraction is *always done in the probe side*, again by measuring the alteration of the SPL in the ear canal due to the stapedial muscle contraction. During the ipsilateral mode, the sound is also presented through the probe, and the AR is measured at the same (ipsilateral) side of the sound stimulation, although the AR in normal ears is occurring in both ears. During the contralateral mode, the sound is presented through the earphone in the opposite (contralateral) side from the probe, while the AR occurring bilaterally is only measured in the probe side.

The AR patterns are interpreted based on the two ways that the AR can be affected by an abnormal process: **sound effect** and **probe effect**. The sound effect simply examines whether the stimulus is loud enough to elicit the AR. Absent/elevated thresholds indicate a possible hearing loss that could prevent sufficient stimulation or possibly indicate a retrocochlear pathology along the auditory nerve. The probe effect examines the efferent pathway of the facial nerve (thus, facial nerve effect), where the abnormality along the facial nerve pathway could prevent the stapedial muscle contraction on the affected side despite the possibility that the sound stimulation is sufficient enough to elicit the AR.

Arbitrary classifications of different AR patterns are shown in Table 2. Type I (normal) is a normal pattern. Type II (sound effect) depicts a "vertical" pattern due to the HL in the affected side. Type III (facial nerve/probe effect) depicts a "diagonal" pattern, where the AR is absent only when the probe is in the affected side. Type IV (conductive effect) depicts a typical pattern where even a unilateral mild CHL could obscure the AR bilaterally.

Acoustic Reflex Patterns

Table 2. Different types (arbitrary classification) of acoustic reflex patterns depending on different pathologies (e.g., the left sides are pathologic in all examples).

Type I: Normal Pattern

	Right	Left
Ipsilateral	Present	Present
Contralateral	Present	Present

Type II: Sound Effect (Retrocochlear Pathology)

	Right	Left
Ipsilateral	Present	*Absent*
Contralateral	Present	*Absent*

Type III: Probe Effect (Facial Nerve Paralysis)

	Right	Left
Ipsilateral	Present	*Absent*
Contralateral	*Absent*	Present

Type IV: Conductive Effect (Unilateral/Bilateral CHL)

	Right	Left
Ipsilateral	*Absent**	*Absent*
Contralateral	*Absent*	*Absent*

*Only unaffected ipsilateral ear in unilateral CHL.

Visual Reinforcement Audiometry (VRA)

(CPT Code: 92579)

It is often not possible to obtain reliable behavioral conditioned responses under earphones from infants, toddlers and children who may exhibit developmental delays and/or physiologic anomalies. **Visual reinforcement audiometry (VRA)** is developed to assess the status of hearing among infants and difficult-to-test populations.

VRA utilizes the principle of **conditioned orientation reflex (COR)** (Suzuki & Ogiba, 1961), where during a conditioning phase, the patient (e.g., infant) is conditioned to the presentation of the auditory stimuli (e.g., warble tones, narrow-band noise, live voice) that are simultaneously presented with intriguing toys inside a transparent lighted box. Once this conditioning is completed at the higher stimulus levels, the test phase can begin with the presentation of the auditory stimuli, followed by the lighting-up of the toy object as soon as the patient turns the head to the direction of the auditory stimuli (Fig. 10). The stimulus presentation levels are then lowered until a reasonably reliable threshold is established. VRA is typically accomplished in sound field using speakers, where **the acquired threshold is an estimate based on the hearing status of the better ear**. However, an insert foam phone can be placed in each ear for more precise measures to assess the hearing status of each ear separately as long as the young infant cooperates and is able to be conditioned.

As lateral sound localization develops at about 6 months of age, VRA is appropriate for infants **from 6 months of age to approximately 2½ to 3 years of age at most**. For older infants, the response characteristics habituate quickly so the audiologist must switch stimuli and/or switch the reinforcer to maintain interest level. For premature infants, the **corrected age** (i.e., chronologic age minus number of weeks the infant was born prematurely) must be considered in the interpretation of the VRA test results.

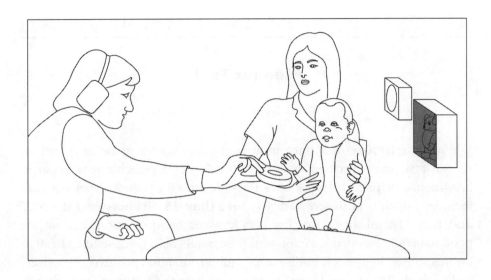

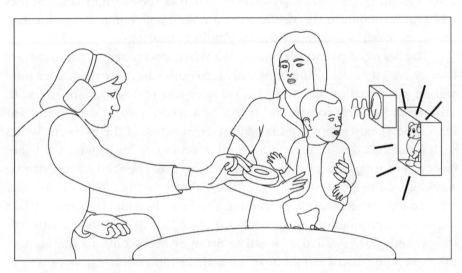

Figure 10. During the VRA, the second examiner inside the audiometric booth (another examiner being outside, controlling the audiometer) is attempting to get the attention of an infant to the center (called "centering") (*top figure*), whereas the infant's head turns toward the sound stimulus presented through a speaker, at the same time the infant is "rewarded" by the lighting-up of the toy (*bottom figure*). Note that the second examiner is wearing an earmuff to "block off" the stimuli presented to eliminate the examiner's bias.

Stenger Test

(CPT Codes: Pure Tone, 92565; Speech, 92577)

When the reliability of a pure tone audiogram seems to be in question, several test procedures are available to rule out a possible **nonorganic** hearing loss or **pseudohypacusis**. Possible cues for pseudohypacusis may include: a significant **discrepancy (more than 15 dB) between the SRT and the PTA**; history involving accidents or compensation; excuse for poor academic performance; or some "unusual" behaviors such as hesitating responses in speech audiometry, numerous false positive responses, and so forth. Traditional behavioral tests such as the **Stenger test** are useful to further confirm the suspicion of a nonorganic component, but they do not necessarily determine the threshold of hearing.

The **Stenger principle** states that when two tones of the same frequency are introduced simultaneously into both ears, only the louder tone will be perceived as one tone. The Stenger test is designed for use with **unilateral hearing losses** and works best when **a large difference (at least 25 dB)** exists between the admitted thresholds of the two ears. When such a difference is observed in a routine pure tone audiogram with various cues of suspicion of nonorganic hearing loss, the Stenger test can be administered by presenting a tone 10 dB above the threshold of the "better" ear and simultaneously presenting a tone at the same frequency 10 dB below the threshold of the "poorer" ear (Martin, 1986). If the patient fails to respond, this is called a **positive Stenger**. According to the Stenger principle, the patient would hear the tone in the poorer ear, because the tone in that ear is perceived as louder than the tone in the better ear. The patient is unaware of the tone in the better ear, but at the same time just doesn't want to admit hearing the tone in the poorer ear. If the patient does respond, this is called a **negative Stenger**. It suggests the absence of nonorganicity as the patient is responding only to the tone that is heard in the admittedly better ear. The patient does not hear the tone in the poorer ear because the hearing loss is real and the tone is below threshold. The Stenger test can be performed with speech stimuli using a similar principle (e.g., spondee words are presented 10 dB above the SRT of the better ear and at the same time 10 dB below the SRT of the poorer ear). As before, no response to spondees would be considered a positive Stenger.

Numerous behavioral tests for pseudohypacusis besides the Stenger test have been developed and are available for clinical use (Martin, 1985). However, their utility is still limited, and the quantification of hearing loss is very poor. Therefore, modern electrophysiologic test techniques such as otoacoustic emissions and auditory brainstem response tests have become widely used to estimate a more precise level of "true" hearing thresholds across different frequencies. Specificity of degree and type of hearing loss and frequency specificity vary among different tests.

Acoustic Reflex (I/C)	Present with near normal or mild HL
Screening TEOAE/DPOAE	Response present with threshold ≤30 dB; Can be affected by middle ear pathology
70/70 DPOAE	Response present with threshold ≤55 dB; Can be affected by middle ear pathology
Threshold ABR	Estimate within 10 to 15 dB of the audiometic thresholds close to near-normal hearing for 2 to 4 kHz; Need tone-burst for more frequency specificity. Differentiate CHL versus SNHL by doing both AC and BC modes
ASSR	Estimate within 10 to 15 dB of the audiometic thresholds for 0.5 to 4 kHz; Variability increases as thresholds become mild to near normal; Differentiate CHL versus SNHL by doing both AC and BC modes

Auditory Brainstem Response (ABR)

(CPT Code: 92585)

As the auditory nerves ascend from the cochlea to the auditory cortex, they pass through different synaptic stations, in a sense, like a switchboard, in order to handle the complexity of auditory signals, such as human speech, which contain complex timing, frequency and intensity cues. At these synaptic stations, physiological potentials are discharged in response to auditory stimulation. The **auditory brainstem response (ABR)**, otherwise called **brainstem evoked auditory response (BEAR)** evaluation, simply attempts to measure these potentials by utilizing electrophysiologic principles similar to those techniques used in EEG and EKG. Electrodes are placed on the head, typically one on the forehead, another on the right mastoid, and a third on the left mastoid (e.g., ipsilateral montage). The sound stimuli, usually clicks, are delivered through either earphones or insert probes placed in each ear. Different stimuli such as tone bursts (e.g., 500 Hz) can also be used to assess more frequency-specific information as the responses obtained using the clicks are typically restricted to the frequency regions between 1000 Hz (Hood, 1998) or even 2000 Hz and 4000 Hz (Bauch & Olson, 1986, 1987; Hall, 1992; van der Drift, Brocaar, & van Zanten, 1987). The stimuli can also be delivered via a BC vibrator to distinguish conductive from sensorineural hearing loss.

Typically, five distinct peaks are elicited in normal human ears with each peak corresponding to the following primary anatomic sites along the brainstem (Moller, Jannetta, & Moller, 1981; Moller & Jannetta, 1985), however, more than one anatomic site is likely contributing to the wave generation (Moore, 1987) (Fig. 11).

Wave I, cochlea/VIIIth nerve (distal);

Wave II, VIIIth nerve (proximal);

Wave III, cochlear nucleus;

Wave IV, superior olivary complex;

Wave V, lateral lemniscus/inferior colliculus

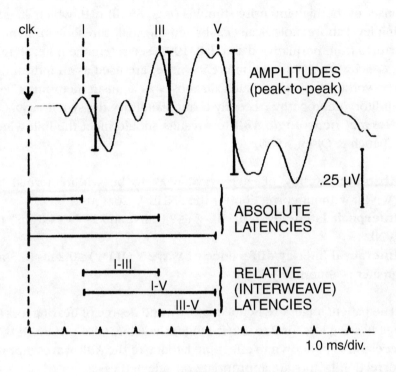

Figure 11. Basic amplitude and latency measures of the ABR adopted from ASHA Audiologic Evaluation Working Group on Auditory Evoked Potential Measurements (Durrant et al., 1988). Terminology is consistent with the classic labeling scheme of Jewett and Williston (1971).

Neurologic ABR Interpretation

The ABR wave peaks occur at precise times (latency), typically within 6 milliseconds (e.g., wave I <2 ms, wave III <4 ms, wave V <6 ms) from the onset of the high-intensity stimulus (e.g., 85 dB nHL which stands for hearing level above biologically calibrated "normal" thresholds). Significant departures from normative data (Hall, 1992, see reference note; Schwartz, Pratt, & Schwartz, 1989, see reference note) are used as an indication for further workup to rule out such diagnoses as acoustic neuroma (Fig. 12) and auditory neuropathy (recently termed auditory dys-synchrony).

   Normal neurologic ABR test results should meet the following criteria (Bauch & Olsen, 1986):

   1. **Absolute latency** of each wave peak to be within normal limits (WNL); Without correction for the SNHL, V ≤6.2 ms.
   2. **Interpeak latencies**, I-III, III-V (≤2.0 ms) and I-V (≤4.0 ms) to be WNL;
   3. **Interaural latency difference of Wave V (ILDv)** ≤0.2 ms (0.3 ms or greater is abnormal!)

   The patient's age, sex, neural maturity, and degree of hearing loss (e.g., average hearing loss for 2 to 4 kHz range) (Bauch & Olsen, 1986, 1987, see referece note) are known to affect the latency of the ABR waves. Appropriate correction factors are appropriate on selected cases.

   The type of hearing loss also influences the wave latencies. A conductive hearing loss, its origin being in the outer or middle ear, affects all wave peaks equally. Thus, the absolute latencies of all waves are delayed with the normal interpeak latencies. An asymmetric SNHL with a possible retro-cochlear etiology (e.g., acoustic neuroma in the internal auditory meatus prior to the level of the cochlear nucleus), on the other hand, typically delays the absolute latencies of waves III and V without the delay of wave I.

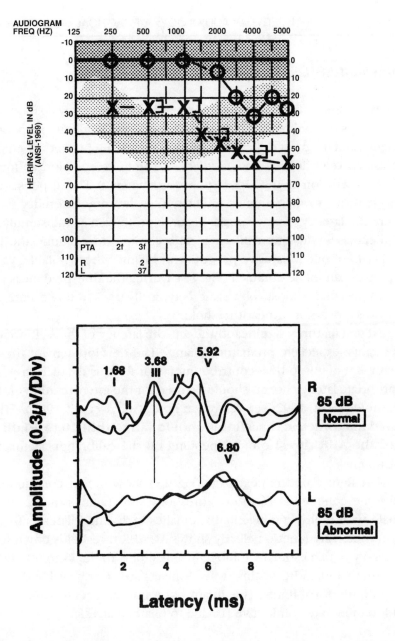

Figure 12. Normal (*R*) and abnormal (*L*) ABR for neurologic evaluation. Wave V latency is significantly delayed for the L (6.80 ms >6.20 ms) with ILDv (0.6 ms) due to a retrocochlear lesion. Note the significant asymmetric SNHL in the audiogram.

Threshold ABR

ABR possesses several advantages over the behavioral evaluation of hearing, such as the audiogram. It does not require any voluntary response from patients, and the most desirable responses are often obtained when patients are asleep (e.g., infants and toddlers may require sedation although the effects of sedation on the ABR response are minimal). The responses are also very sensitive to the stimulus intensity (i.e., **latency-intensity function** where the latency of wave peaks become prolonged as the stimulus intensity decreases), making ABR an ideal technique to examine the hearing level (HL) of uncooperative patients and infants where reliable, voluntary responses cannot be obtained (Fig. 13). During the threshold measures, the wave V peak stays most robust and is typically tracked down until it eventually disappears at or near threshold.

Neural maturity significantly affects the latency of the ABR wave peaks for infants, especially premature infants. The development of the myelin sheath is thought to be a contributing factor for this delay. Therefore, age-appropriate latency norms should be used for the interpretation of the ABR thresholds (Hall, 1992, see reference note; Gorga et al., 1987). **The estimated audiometric thresholds should fall within 10 to 15 dB better than the ABR thresholds**, depending on the calibration factor of each instrument.

The figures on the next page (Fig. 13) show the air conduction (*top*) and bone conduction (*bottom*) threshold ABR tracings of a 2-month-old female with multiple congenital anomalies including bilateral atresia. The latency-intensity function clearly shows AC ABR thresholds down to 60 dB bilaterally which estimate audiogram thresholds to be 45 to 50 dB HL. On the other hand, in BC testing, wave V peaks are clearly visible down to 20 dB, within normal limits. This infant has a normal cochlear function with mild to moderate conductive HL due to bilateral atresia.

Air Conduction Threshold ABR Tracings

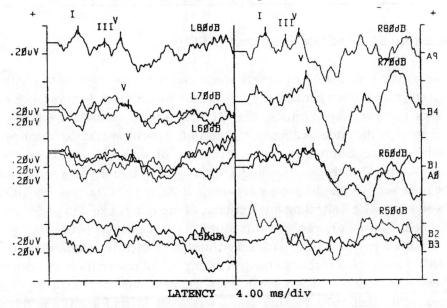

LATENCY   4.00 ms/div

Bone Conduction Threshold ABR Tracings

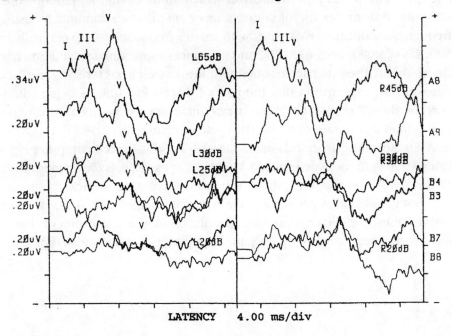

LATENCY   4.00 ms/div

Figure 13. ABR tracings for a 2-month-old with multiple congenital anomalies.

Auditory Steady-State Response (ASSR)

Due to the very nature of neural synchronization, the most robust ABR waveforms are often generated by a stimulus with a short duration such as clicks. However, the shortness of the clicks in turn produces a spread of energy over the wide frequency regions of the cochlear (i.e., basilar membrane). Consequently, frequency specificity of the click has been the "Achilles heel" of the ABR technique, because the ABR allows a threshold estimate only for the frequency region of 2000 to 4000 Hz, possibly 1000 to 4000 Hz. The ABR using low-frequency tone bursts like 250 or 500 Hz has been utilized to overcome this problem (Gorga et al., 2006).

An alternative to the ABR called **auditory steady state response (ASSR)** testing has recently emerged after years of research efforts (Cone-Wesson et al., 2002; Davis & Hirsh, 1976; Dobie & Wilson, 1995; Galambos et al., 1981; Hall, 1979; Picton et al., 2002). ASSR differs from ABR in three different ways: (1) stimulus characteristics; (2) response characteristics; and (3) response analysis. Unlike ABR which utilizes a transient *on-off* stimulus, the ASSR makes use of continuous or *steady-state* stimulus by using frequency-modulated (FM) tones with carrier frequencies (CF) clinically at 500, 1000, 2000, and 4000 Hz, and generates the estimated audiometric thresholds at these carrier frequencies. Response characteristics are thus based on the assumption that the part of the cochlea that is being stimulated by the CF (e.g., 1000 Hz) must be intact for the cochlea to respond to the modulation rate (e.g., 80 Hz, cycle of change in the CF) producing an ASSR. Response analysis is made through a sophisticated computer algorithm to analyze the synchronized ASSR that, in essence, is *the synchronous EEG responses* in the brain; thus there is no wave peak to pick!

Both ABR and ASSR have their own advantages and disadvantages (Table 3). Each clinician, therefore, should develop a test protocol that is most appropriate depending on patient population and clinic setup.

Table 3. Comparison of the features for ABR and ASSR

	ABR	ASSR
WNL:	Accurate estimation	May overestimate
Test time:	Relatively fast	Needs more time
State:	Sleep or awake	Very quiet state
Infant:	Sleep-deprived or sedation	Sedation required
Anesthesia:	Fairly robust	OK for higher modulation
Electrodes:	Typically three	Three; different locations
Invasiveness:	Noninvasive	Noninvasive
Ear-specific:	Yes; Test one ear	Yes; Test binaurally
Freq-specific:	Need tone burst	500 to 4000 Hz
Degree:	Up to moderate/severe	Severe or greater degree
Type:	Yes; AC versus BC	Yes; AC versus BC
BC:	Yes; Masking not required	Yes; Masking required
CHL:	Delay of latencies	Elevated thresholds
Neural dysfunction:	Yes; IPL, CM	Not distinguish HL versus AN
Availability:	Widely available	Yes, but somewhat limited

WNL = within normal limits; AC = air conduction; BC = bone conduction; CHL = conductive hearing loss; IPL = interpeak latency; CM = cochlear microphonics; HL = hearing loss; AN = auditory neuropathy/dys-synchrony.

Electrocochleography (ECoG)

(CPT Code: 92584)

Electrophysiologic components measured during electrocochleography (ECoG) are essentially the same as ABR except that in ECoG the wave I component is analyzed more closely. ECoG measures are specifically designed to identify electrophysiologic signs of Ménière's disease (Coats, 1981, 1986). In an ECoG evaluation, the subcomponents of wave I are referred to as **summating potential (SP)** and **action potential (AP)**, both of which are known to be generated within the cochlea (Fig. 14). In fact, AP should be considered as synonymous to wave I of ABR. In comparing the amplitudes of SP and AP among normal patients and Ménière's patients, the SP amplitude as compared to the AP amplitude (i.e., SP/AP ratio) is known to be significantly elevated among patients with Ménière's disease and has been hypothetically associated with endolymphatic hydrops (excessive accumulation of endolymph within the cochlea). Using a conservative criterion, **an amplitude ratio of SP over AP greater than 0.5 (50%) is typically considered to be significant**, that is, a positive indication for Ménière's disease. A positive ECoG finding is found in only 60% of Ménière's patients. Thus, while the sensitivity of ECoG for Ménière's disease is relatively high, the specificity is low, that is, a negative ECoG does not sufficiently rule out the diagnosis of Ménière's disease.

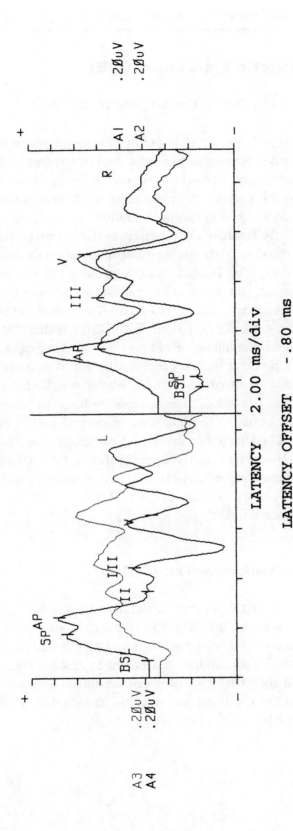

Figure 14. Elevated SP/AP ratio (0.91) in the left ear as compared to normal SP/AP ratio (0.08) identified in the right ear. The SP/AP ratio is much greater than 0.5 in the left ear and a positive indication for Ménière's disease. The absolute latency of AP (*horizontal axis*) is consistent across all waveforms, whereas the amplitudes of the AP and SP (*vertical axis*) vary greatly across the waveforms, which are typical of ECoG and ABR recordings. Also note that absolute latencies of waves I (AP), III and V, and interpeak latencies I–III, III–V, and I–V are all within normal limits bilaterally with respect to the neurologic ABR.

Otoacoustic Emissions (OAE)

(CPT Codes: Limited, 92587; Comprehensive, 92588)

Otoacoustic emission (OAE) (Kemp, 1978) is a fairly new technique in the field of audiology, but its value is becoming more and more relevant in differential diagnosis of hearing loss. Normal human ears, specifically **outer hair cells (OHC)** within the cochlea, have the capacity to emit sounds (i.e., "emissions,") upon auditory stimulation. A unique characteristic of OAE lies in the fact that **only healthy OHC generate these emissions**. Almost 99% of the time, the OAE is absent from impaired ears with more than a mild degree of hearing loss. Thus, the simple presence or absence of the OAE across frequencies can separate normal ears from those with some degree of hearing loss **greater than 25 to 30 dB**. Two common OAE tests are **transient-evoked OAE (TEOAE)** and **distortion-product OAE (DPOAE)**. Both procedures are noninvasive and very quick, requiring only the simple placement of a probe at the ear canal entrance, and essentially provide equivalent information. Because of these advantages, OAE tests have become very common procedures for neonatal hearing screening. However, precaution must be taken to make sure of normal middle ear function as OAE results can be affected by middle ear pathology (e.g., fluid presence, ETD) (Amedee, 1995; Marshall, Heller, & Westhusin, 1997; Owens et al., 1993; Tilanus, Van Stenis, & Snik, 1995). The OAE response can be obscured in middle ears with fluid more than 60% of the time (Koike & Wetmore, 1999, see reference note).

Transient-Evoked Otoacoustic Emissions (TEOAE)

TEOAE uses a click stimulus that is set at a default level of around 95 dB peak SPL to elicit emissions from OHC (Fig. 15). Like a click stimulus for ABR, the frequency spectrum of the stimulus becomes rather broad due to its short duration. Thus, the clicks produce movement in a broad area of the basilar membrane and the OHC responses can be obtained and analyzed from 1000 Hz to 5000 Hz. Frequency-specific information is still observed in 1000 Hz intervals within this frequency range.

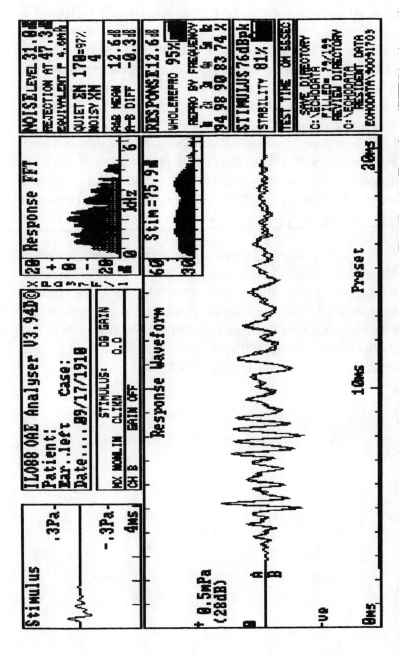

Figure 15. Normal TEOAE generated by ILO88 OAE Analyzer. "Response in Fast Fourier Transform (FFT)" is shown in dark shadow just above "stimulus FFT" of a click stimulus (*see top left*). An oscilloscopic "response waveform" shows high-frequency components generated at the basal end and earlier in time than low-frequency components generated at the apical end of the cochlear. "Reproduction rates by frequency (i.e., 1 to 5 kHz)" are indicated in percentage, and should be greater than 50% for each frequency to be considered a reproducible response. "Test time" (*lower right*) shows that the entire test took only 55 seconds to complete for the left ear.

Distortion-Product Otoacoustic Emissions (DPOAE)

DPOAE uses two stimulus tones (F1 and F2) to stimulate the basilar membrane in close proximity, resulting in a distortion tone somewhere between these two tones, typically in the frequency region of 2F1 to F2 (Gorga et al., 1993; Kemp, 1997) (Fig. 16). DPOAE technique captures the emissions that are produced at the point of this distortion tone. Optimal combinations of two frequencies and their intensity levels have been studied extensively to be incorporated into commercially available DPOAE equipment.

In advanced applications of DPOAE, the levels of two stimulus tones can be varied from 65/55 dB (for F1 and F2 frequencies, respectively) to 70/70 dB. The lower stimulus levels are used to rule out a mild degree of hearing loss ($\leq$25 dB) (Gorga et al, 1993; Gorga et al, 1997), whereas the higher stimulus levels are used to rule out a moderate hearing loss ($\leq$55 dB) (Gorga et al., 2003).

Research efforts have also been made to estimate audiometric thresholds from OAE data (Boege & Janssen, 2002; Gorga et al., 1997; Gorga et al., 2003; Kummer, Janssen, & Arnold, 1998). However, data have not yielded a precise correlation to "predict" a certain pure tone threshold value within reasonable proximity, other than general pass/fail criteria described above. For example, a distortion product (DP) level of 19 dB would not be correlated to a certain pure tone threshold value, say 25 dB HL.

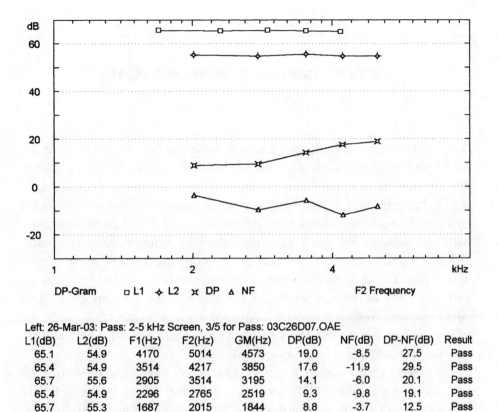

Left: 26-Mar-03: Pass: 2-5 kHz Screen, 3/5 for Pass: 03C26D07.OAE

L1(dB)	L2(dB)	F1(Hz)	F2(Hz)	GM(Hz)	DP(dB)	NF(dB)	DP-NF(dB)	Result
65.1	54.9	4170	5014	4573	19.0	-8.5	27.5	Pass
65.4	54.9	3514	4217	3850	17.6	-11.9	29.5	Pass
65.7	55.6	2905	3514	3195	14.1	-6.0	20.1	Pass
65.4	54.9	2296	2765	2519	9.3	-9.8	19.1	Pass
65.7	55.3	1687	2015	1844	8.8	-3.7	12.5	Pass

Figure 16. DP-gram depicting typical DPOAE responses generated in a 65/55 screening paradigm, meeting "Pass" criteria for all frequencies from 2 through 5 kHz. To be considered as "Pass," DP level has to be no worse than − 6 dB and DP-NP should be greater than 6 dB.

Central Auditory Processing (CAP)

(CPT Code: 92620)

Despite the presence of normal hearing, some individuals complain of difficulty understanding normally spoken conversation. The difficulty is often more noticeable in noisy situations and when more than one person is talking at the same time. Complaints are more common among school-aged children than adults because the CAP disorder (CAPD) is often associated with and could be a cause of learning delays, including reading and math, or speech and language delay, academic underachievement, or attention deficit (Fig. 17). However, adults can certainly exhibit a CAPD or grow up with one without being identified. A sample checklist for suspected CAPD could include: Problems understanding someone who talks fast; problems following instructions; confuses words with similar sound (e.g., six for fix); trouble paying attention in background noise.

A typical CAP evaluation may include speech discrimination of muffled words (e.g., Filtered Word Test), in noise (e.g., Auditory Figure Ground), or repetition of multiple words (e.g., Competing Words Test) or sentences (e.g., Competing Sentences Test) spoken at the same time. A percentile score of each subtest is compared against normative data among specific age groups (Keith, 1986).

Examples of Filtered Words Subtest

own, leave, you, on, may

Examples of Auditory Figure-Ground Subtest

all, back, end, take, coat

Examples of Competing Words Subtest

waste (R)/cage (L), need (R)/case (L), may (R)/them (L)

Examples of Competing Sentences Subtest

The floor looked clean (R)./The man came early (L).
The dinner plate is hot (R)./The lady ate a pear (L).

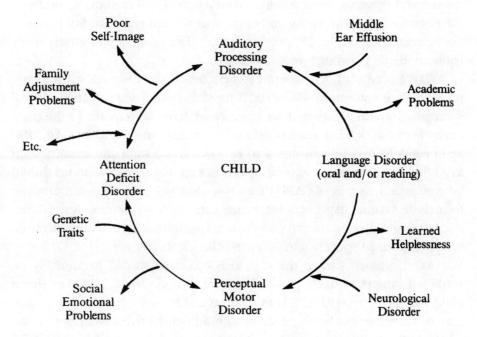

Figure 17. A model of possible factors contributing to a child's performance problems (adapted from Keith, 1986). In this model, auditory processing disorders are considered to result from a number of possible causes, including neurologic disorders and genetic traits, and from early and frequent middle ear effusion. The model treats auditory processing disorders as one of many factors that should be considered when evaluating children who are having difficulty achieving their potential. The model also includes some of the consequences of developmental disorders.

CAPD Intervention

Remediation may include preferential seating or even use of an auditory trainer, and various other steps (Fig. 18). However, children with CAPD often exhibit a variety of problems in a wide range of areas, for example, speech and language, or academics such as math and reading, resulting in the need for help with social and emotional adjustment in addition to academic remediation (Fig. 17, previous page). Therefore, a multidisciplinary team approach is strongly recommended.

CAPD is typically considered to be a functional disorder without any physiologic involvement. However, if basic audiometric evaluations reveal some abnormal findings such as absence of acoustic reflexes in the presence of normal hearing, further diagnostic evaluations including OAE, ABR, and even MRI may be warranted to rule out any central abnormality such as auditory neuropathy, and referral to other appropriate disciplines should be considered. As part of CAPD diagnosis, some investigators even propose to include various psychoacoustic measures such as masking level differences, rapidly altering speech perception, synthetic sentence identification, time-compressed speech, and so forth (Musiek, 1985).

As mentioned earlier, the diagnosis of CAPD should presumably be made with the presence of normal hearing. It is common, however, that a child who is referred for CAPD evaluation and having a problem at school, may be diagnosed as having a slight to mild conductive loss either in one ear or both ears due to multiple ear infections. Some children may even have a sensorineural hearing loss that has not been identified. Children with a peripheral hearing loss, either conductive or sensorineural in nature, are likely to exhibit "processing" deficits because of the very presence of peripheral hearing loss even if minimal in degree (Bess, 1985; Tharpe & Bess, 1999). The peripheral hearing loss must be treated according to standard protocols such as medication and bilateral ventilation tubes for otitis media or amplification for the case of sensorineural hearing loss.

UNDERSTANDING AUDITORY PROCESSING

Your child was just evaluated for his/her ability to process speech in a difficult listening environment. This is known as *Central Auditory Processing*. Quite simply, this is more like a test of "listening ability" than like a test of "hearing ability". During this test, your child must be able to repeat what is said on a tape against background noise or competing words. If your child is found to be weak in performing this type of listening task, we suggest the following for improving his/her performance:

1. Classroom placement. (Avoid seating child in settings that are noisy or reverberant and avoid open classroom placement).

2. Request preferential seating near place where teacher spends most of his/her time giving auditory instruction and away from distracting auditory and visual noise.

3. Teach your child to use visual information (look and listen).

4. Encourage teacher(s) to gain your child's attention before giving auditory instruction.

5. Rephrase or restate important information to provide auditory redundancy.

6. Give your child time to think and time to respond to auditory instruction and/or questions.

7. Use verbal devices for getting your child's attention, such as calling his/her name and saying "listen" and/or "are you ready" before making assignments.

8. Limit the amount of information in each instruction.

Any remedial program should not only arrange for the management of the child but also recognize the child's own responsibility in his/her own remediation. When children learn to take care of their own needs through better organization, i.e. asking for repetition, double checking assignments, and other self-help behavior; better academic success and improvement in self-image is achieved.

Should you have any further questions, please contact the Audiology Clinic located in the Physician Office Center at (304) 598-4825.

{Recommendations adapted from a screening test manual for *Auditory Processing Disorders* written by Robert W. Keith, 1986}

Figure 18. A summary of possible recommendations for children with CAPD. (Adapted with permission from Keith, R. W. [1986]. *SCAN: A screening test for auditory processing disorders.* San Diego, CA: Harcourt Brace Jovanovich. Copyright 1986 by Harcourt Brace Jovanovich.)

PART II

Evaluation of
Balance Disorders

Evaluation and treatment of dizzy patients seem to vary depending on which discipline of medicine from which a patient seeks an opinion regarding his/her symptoms. In an otolaryngology clinic, hearing and the vestibular system (Fig. 19) are commonly evaluated to rule out the inner ear as the origin of dizziness and imbalance.

In Part I, evaluation of hearing disorders has been described. In Part II, one of the most common evaluation procedures for dizzy patients, called electronystagmography (ENG), will be described in detail. A history is also critical in diagnosis of dizzy patients. The Dizziness Handicap Inventory (DHI) is described as one systematic way to obtain a detailed history. Rotational Chair Test and Computerized Dynamic Posturography (CDP) may be included as a part of a more comprehensive evaluation of dizzy patients. The Clinical Test of Sensory Interaction on Balance (CTSIB) can provide further information and is useful as part of vestibular rehabilitation.

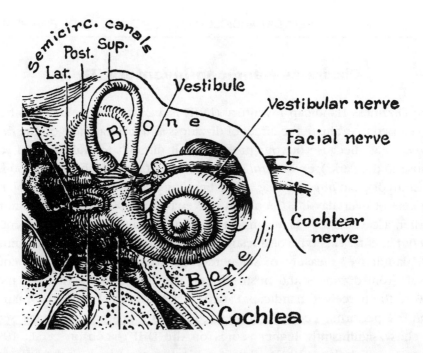

Figure 19. An enlarged cross-sectional view of the vestibular system that is one of the main organs for balance (Brodel, 1946). (From Brodel, M. [1946] *Three unpublished drawings of the anatomy of the human ear*. Philadelphia, PA: W.B. Saunders. Copyright 1946 by W.B. Saunders. Reprinted with permission.)

Dizziness Handicap Inventory (DHI)

The Dizziness Handicap Inventory (DHI) is a 25-item scale that has been developed to evaluate the effect of dizziness and unsteadiness on the *functional* (e.g., Because of your problem, is it difficult to walk around your house in the dark?), *emotional* (e.g., Because of your problem, do you feel frustrated?), and *physical* (e.g., Does bending over increase your problem?) aspects of everyday life (Jacobson & Newman, 1990) (Fig. 20). As noted earlier, a case history is an important part of diagnosis and treatment of dizzy patients. This type of questionnaire can assist clinicians in obtaining a "quantitative" measure of self-perceived disability-handicap that could result from dizziness and unsteadiness. The higher the score, the more severe the perceived handicap. Patients with abnormal Sensory Organization Test performance on Computerized Dynamic Posturography also seem to show significantly higher scores on the DHI (Jacobson et al., 1991; Robertson & Ireland, 1995). Thus, a subjective scale such as the DHI, may shed more insight into how patients are functioning in the "real-world," where sensory input from the vestibular system needs to be integrated with visual and proprioceptive input.

The DHI could be further used as pre- and post-test to determine the effectiveness of vestibular rehabilitation (Brown et al., 2001; Cohen & Kimball, 2003; Krebs et al., 1993; Mruzek et al., 1995). A less time-consuming screening version of the DHI (DHI-S) has also been developed for clinics, such as a primary care office (Jacobson & Calder, 1998).

WVU Department of Otolaryngology

Dizziness Handicap Inventory

Instructions: The purpose of this scale is to identify difficulties that you may be experiencing because of your dizziness or unsteadiness. Please answer "yes," "no," or "sometimes" to each question. *Answer each question as it pertains to your dizziness or unsteadiness problem.*

	Yes	Sometimes	No
1. Does looking up increase your problem?			
2. Because of your problem, do you feel frustrated?			
3. Because of your problem, do you restrict your travel for business or recreation?			
4. Does walking down the aisle of a supermarket increase your problem?			
5. Because of your problem, do you have difficulty getting into and out of bed?			
6. Does your problem significantly restrict your participation in social activities such as going out to dinner, going to movies, dancing or parties?			
7. Because of your problem, do you have difficulty reading?			
8. Does performing more ambitious activities like sports, dancing, household chores such as sweeping or putting dishes away, increase your problem?			
9. Because of your problem, are you afraid to leave your homw without having someone accompany you?			
10. Because of your problem, have you been embarrassed in front of others?			
11. Do quick movements of your head increase your problem?			
12. Because of your problem, do you avoid heights?			
13. Does turning over in bed increase your problem?			
14. Because of your problem, is it difficult for you to do strenuous housework or yardwork?			
15. Because of your problem, do you think people may think you are intoxicated?			
16. Because of your problem, is it difficult for you to go for a walk by yourself?			
17. Does walking down a sidewalk increase your problem?			
18. Because of your problem, is it difficult for you to concentrate?			
19. Because of your problem, is it difficult for you to walk around your house in the dark?			
20. Because of your problem, are you afraid to stay home alone?			
21. Because of your problem, do you feel handicapped?			
22. Has your problem placed stress on your relationships with members of your family or friends?			
23. Because of your problem, are you depressed?			
24. Does your problem interfere with your job or household responsibilities?			
25. Does bending over increase your pain?			

Figure 20. The **Dizziness Handicap Inventory (DHI)** is designed to examine self-perceived impact of dizziness and unsteadiness on a patient's quality of life. Each item of a 25-item scale receives 4 points for *yes*, 2 points for *sometimes*, and 0 points for *no*, and a score of zero indicates minimal impact while the higher score indicates an increasing impact on the patient's well-being.

Electronystagmography (ENG)

(CPT Codes: 92541 through 92545)

Electronystagmography is an electrophysiologic test for peripheral vestibular end organs and for central integration of neural centers of the balance mechanism. Actual electrode measures are monitored through the patient's eye movements, utilizing the electrical potential around the eye called the corneoretinal potential.

When the patient has a vertiginous attack, it is associated with quick, jerky movements of the eyeballs called **nystagmus**. In fact, the ENG is the only recordable documentation of nystagmus as a sign of vertigo (Fig. 21).

In recent years, the process to record eyeball movements through electrodes has been replaced by infrared technology where an actual video image of the eyeballs can be visualized, traced, and saved on a computer. Thus, the ENG is now referred to as **videonystagmography (VNG)** to reflect this change. However, the traditionally used subtests and their interpretation still remain the same.

ENG/VNG typically consists of a series of subtests as follows:

1. **Saccade Test**
2. **Tracking (Pursuit) Test**
3. **Gaze Test**
4. **Positional Test**
5. **Optokinetic Test**
6. **Dix-Hallpike Maneuver**
7. **Caloric Test**

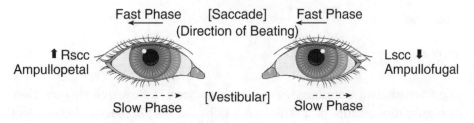

RIGHT BEATING NYSTAGMUS
(Rotating to the Right; RW; LC)

Fast Phase   [Saccade]   Fast Phase
(Direction of Beating)

↑ Rscc   Lscc ↓
Ampullopetal   Ampullofugal

- - - →   [Vestibular]   - - - →
Slow Phase   Slow Phase

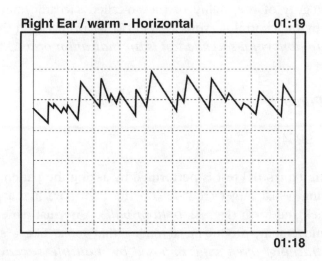

Right Ear / warm - Horizontal   **01:19**

01:18

Figure 21. An example of "right-beating" nystagmus. The direction of the beat is associated with the fast phase of the eyeball movement and depicted as the upward line on the recording. The upward direction on the vertical axis of the graph indicates Rightward movement; the downward direction indicates the leftward movement. The right-beating nystagmus may be observed when the head is rotating to the right or during the right-warm (RW) or left-cool (LC) irrigations of the caloric testing.

Saccade

(CPT Code: 92541)

The **saccade** test examines the patient's ability to follow quickly direction-changing movements of a target on a light bar that is placed about 4 feet in front of the patient, typically in a sitting up-position (Fig. 22, *top half*).

The integrity of the ability of the so-called saccadic mechanism is maintained by the central nervous system (CNS), primarily in the cerebellum. Thus, *an abnormal saccade test is an indication of a CNS disorder.*

Tracking (Pursuit)

(CPT Code: 92545)

The **tracking (pursuit)** test is performed by asking the patient to follow a slow-moving visual target (red dot on the light bar) like a pendulum swinging back and forth (Fig. 22, *bottom half*). A normal patient follows the target movement, producing a tracing that looks like a sine wave. *Abnormal tracking, often superimposed by **multiple saccades**, is an indication of a CNS disorder.*

You can also perform the tracking test during a physical exam by moving a finger or pencil slowly back and forth in front of the patient's face. You should observe smooth movement of the eyes without any jerky pauses.

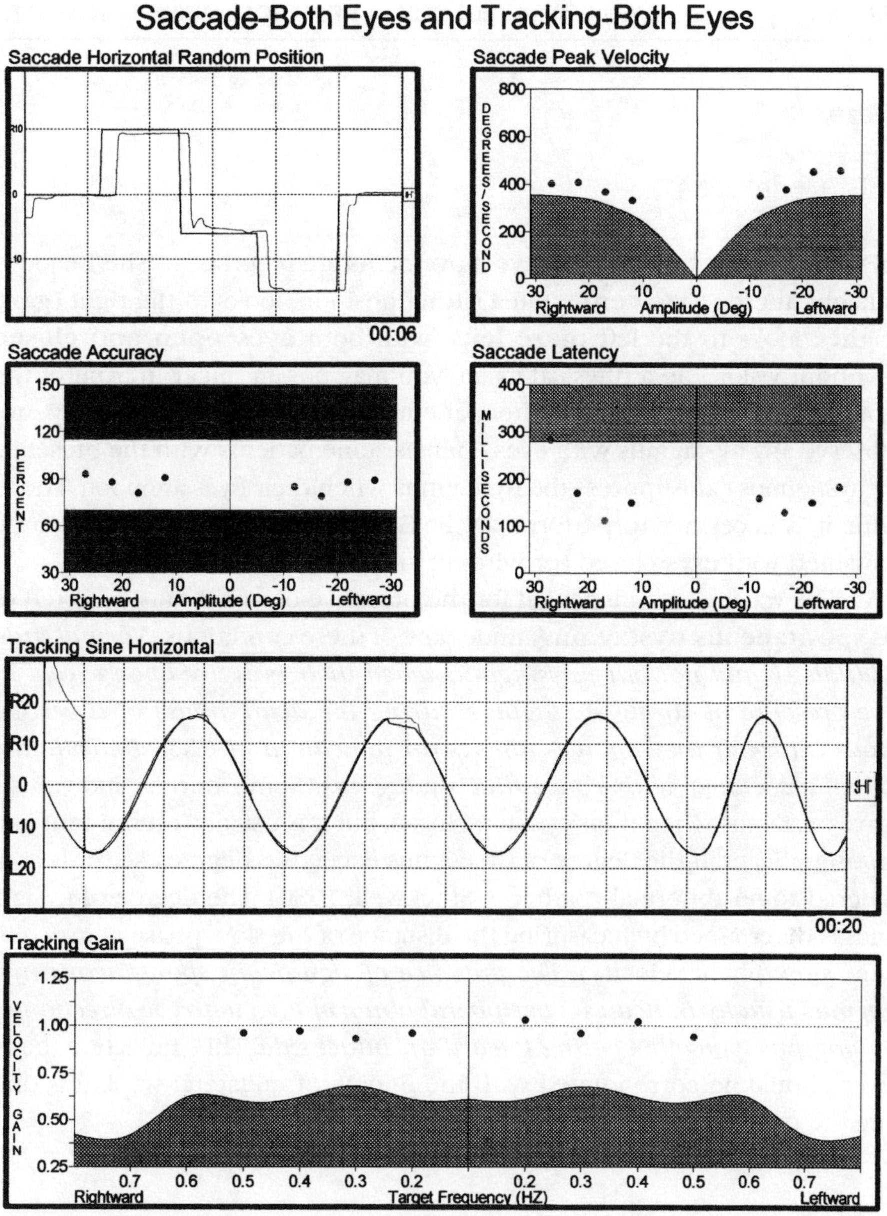

Saccade-Both Eyes and Tracking-Both Eyes

Figure 22. Normal saccade tracing (*top half*) with all the criteria (position, peak velocity, accuracy, and latency) being within normal range (outside of the shaded area). Also shown (*bottom half*) is a normal tracking depicted by a smooth sine wave and tracking gain within normal range (above the shaded area).

Gaze

(CPT Code: 92541)

In the **gaze** test, the patient's eye movements are recorded as she/he looks straight ahead (**gaze center**) in a sitting position, looks to the right (**gaze right**), looks to the left (**gaze left**), with both **eyes open and closed** (without vision). In a physical exam, you may pose a finger in front of the patient's face and observe the patient's eyes; however, you may not observe any nystagmus with eyes open as some patients with the presence of nystagmus can suppress the nystagmus when their eyes are open. Therefore, it is necessary to perform the ENG/VNG where the tracings can be obtained with eyes closed (or without vision during VNG) (Fig. 23).

The tracings are inspected for the presence of nystagmus (referred to as **spontaneous nystagmus**) under any of these conditions. *Normal individuals should not have nystagmus when their eyes are open except in the presence of strong nystagmus during the acute phase of a vertiginous attack. If they do, it is always an indication of CNS abnormality, often associated with congenital nystagmus.* Some normal individuals have nystamus when their eyes are closed, but it is usually intermittent and not significant. If the degree of nystagmus exceeds 6 degrees/sec, it is considered to be abnormal (Barber & Stockwell, 1980). The degree of nystagmus is determined by measuring the distance of the slow phase per second (i.e., slow phase velocity). *The presence of significant spontaneous nystagmus usually indicates a peripheral abnormality, with the direction of nystagmus typically beating toward an intact side.* This indication, however, should be corroborated with the finding of unilateral weakness during the caloric testing.

Gaze - Both Eyes

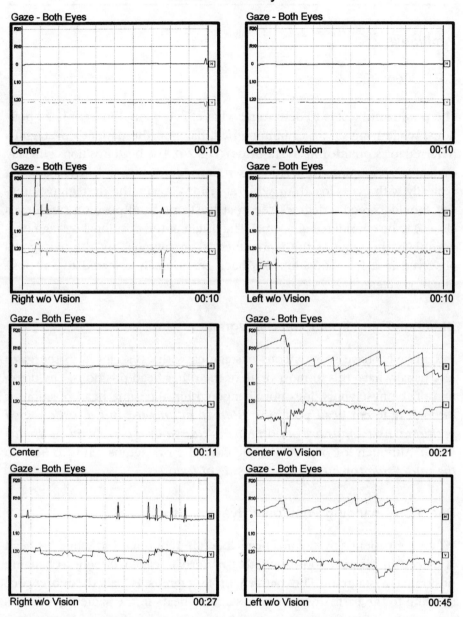

Figure 23. Normal gaze (*top half*) without any significant nystagmus (*top line, horizontal channel; bottom line, vertical channel in each condition*), whereas abnormal gaze is shown in the bottom half with significant spontaneous nystagmus with slow-phase velocity (SPV) greater than 6 degrees being observed in center and left-gaze positions.

Positional

(CPT Code: 92542)

The **positional** test is to determine what effect, if any, different head positions, while lying on an examining bed, have on the patient's nystagmus (referred to as **positional nystagmus**) (Fig. 24). The head positions typically evaluated are supine, right-side down, left-side down, and head hanging, typically with eyes closed (or without vision). Again, the nystagmus intensity should exceed 6 degrees/sec in at least one head position (with eyes closed) to be considered abnormal. The origin of the positional nystagmus is essentially the same as the "spontaneous" nystagmus, but the nystagmus observed in a lying position has been traditionally referred to as "positional" nystagmus.

Direction-Fixed Positional Nystagmus

Patients who have spontaneous nystagmus with eyes closed in the **gaze** test, usually have this in most or all of the other head positions. The direction of the nystagmus does not change within the same head position or through different head positions. *Both spontaneous and direction-fixed positional nystagmus are almost always caused by a peripheral vestibular lesion.* Although it is not always the case, the nystagmus tends to *beat to the intact side (or away from the side of lesion)*.

Direction-Changing Positional Nystagmus

When the patient's nystagmus beats in a different direction while his head is placed in different positions, this pattern is called direction-changing positional nystagmus. The pattern of nystagmus is called "**geotropic**" (beating to the earth) when the nystagmus beats in the same direction as the ear that is in the down position (e.g., right-beating nystagmus with right-ear-down or left-beating nystagmus with left-ear down). The pattern is called "**ageotropic**" (beating away from the earth) when the nystagmus beats in the opposite direction, that is, right beating with the left-ear down, left beating with the right-ear down. The geotropic pattern is often associated with a peripheral lesion whereas the ageotropic pattern is typically associated with a CNS lesion. *If the nystagmus changes direction in a single head position, it is always of CNS origin.*

Positional Nystagmus Test

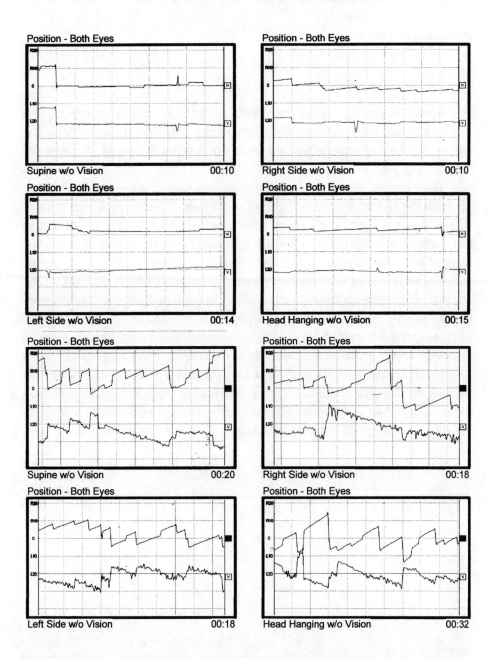

Figure 24. Normal positional test without any significant positional nystagmus (*straight line, top half*) in all "stationary" head positions and abnormal positional test with significant left-beating direction-fixed nystagmus (*bottom half*) in all positions, usually beating toward the intact side (*top line, horizontal channel; bottom line, vertical channel in each condition*).

Optokinetic (OPK)

(CPT Code: 92544)

The **optokinetic** test is performed by asking the patient to watch a series of fast-moving red light dots moving to the right and then the left. The speed of the dots may be altered from 20 degrees/sec to 40 degrees/sec (Fig. 25, *top half*).

The optokinetic stimulus provokes nystagmus beating in the direction opposite to the movement of the dots. For example, "optokinetic right" will produce a left-beating nystagmus. The eyes follow the movement of the fast-moving light dots (smooth pursuit), which corresponds to the slow-phase component of the optokinetic tracings, while the saccadic adjustment is depicted as the fast phase component, which determines, by definition, the direction of the nystagmus. In a normal patient, the intensity of optokinetic nystagmus is the same for rightward or leftward moving dots, respectively. *An asymmetry of the responses and/or a degraded response with a faster moving simulus (Fig. 25, bottom half), is an abnormal indication, suggesting a CNS disorder,* which could be similar to abnormalities in saccade (optokinetic fast component) and/or pursuit (optokinetic slow component) tests because both of these mechanisms are involved in the optokinetic test paradigm (Baloh & Honrubia, 2001).

Optokinetic - Both Eyes

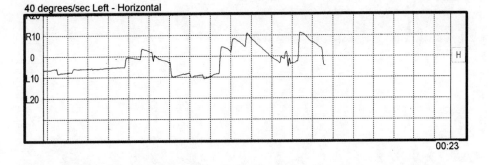

Figure 25. Normal optokinetic (OPK) tracings (*top half*) with slow phase velocity (SPV) consistent with the speed of the dots (e.g., 20 degrees versus 40 degrees) without any asymmetry and abnormal OPK (*bottom half*) with significantly degraded SPV where the patient could not maintain OPK velocity at the higher speed (i.e., 40 degrees).

Dix-Hallpike Maneuver

(CPT Code: With recording, 92542; Without recording, 92532)

The **Dix-Hallpike** maneuver is a test that is useful in diagnosing a specific disorder, namely, **benign paroxysmal positional vertigo (BPPV).** It is performed by briskly laying the patient back, so that the head is hanging over one shoulder, watching the eyes, returning the patient to the sitting position, and again watching the eyes (Fig. 26). The maneuver is then repeated with the patient's head hanging over the other shoulder. A positive response is observed as horizontal **rotary nystagmus** that appears after the patient has been laid backward. It may appear when the patient's head is hanging over the right shoulder, the left shoulder, or both.

The characteristics of this nystagmus are:

1. Delayed for a few seconds in onset;
2. Transient;
3. Accompanied by vertigo;
4. Fatigable, meaning that if a positive response is observed on the first maneuver, the maneuver should be repeated and the response is definitely weaker the second time.

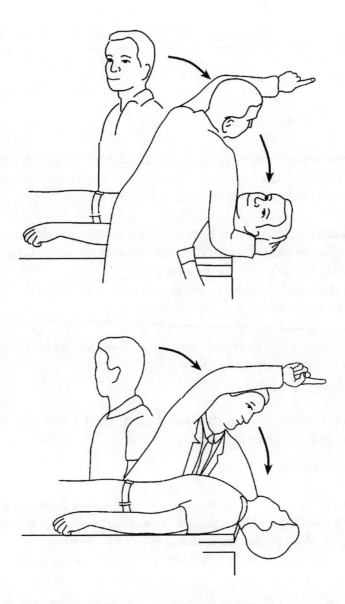

Figure 26. Dix-Hallpike maneuver for inducing paroxysmal positional nystagmus. Patient is moved rapidly from the sitting to head-hanging position, with the left-ear-downward maneuver (*top*) or the right-ear-downward maneuver (*bottom*).

Caloric

(CPT Code: 92543)

The **caloric** test is performed by irrigating each of the patient's ear canals with both **warm** and **cool** water (Fig. 27). The standard water temperature is 30 degrees centigrade for the cool irrigation and 40 degrees centigrade for the warm.

During the test, the patient is placed supine with eyes closed (or without vision) and **head raised by 30 degrees** to place the **lateral (horizontal) semicircular canals** into the vertical plane.

The direction of elicited nystagmus differs according to the ear and the irrigation temperature as follows (COWS):

C—**Cold** water inhibits the lateral canal of the irrigated ear and causes nystagmus beating toward

O—the **Opposite** side.

W—**Warm** water excites the lateral canal of the irrigated ear and causes nystagmus beating toward

S—the **Same** ear.

The intensity of a caloric response is determined by finding the point at which the intensity of the response is maximal and then measuring and averaging the **slow-phase velocities (SPV)** of a few nystagmus beats around the peak. The calculation of the SPV is typically done automatically by a computer.

Caloric - Both Eyes

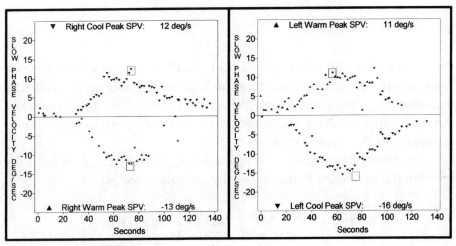

Caloric Weakness: 4% in the right ear

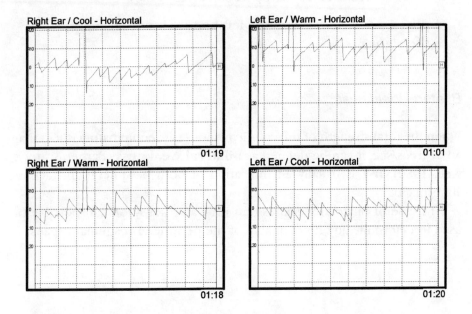

Figure 27. Normal caloric test results showing reasonably symmetric caloric responses from both sides, depicted by rounded liplike shapes on both sides. Each dot (called pod, *top figure*) corresponds to a single nystagmus shown in the bottom graph in each of the four conditions (e.g., right ear cool, left ear cool, right ear warm, left ear warm).

Unilateral Weakness

One of the most significant findings in ENG/VNG is the **unilateral weakness**, where caloric responses from one ear are significantly weaker than the other (Fig. 28). A significant UW is a very useful finding for the otologist as it often localizes the lesion to the ear (i.e., peripheral vestibular system) with the weaker response.

The UW is calculated by comparing the caloric strength of each ear, dividing the difference between ears by the total strength:

$$UW = \frac{(RW + RC) - (LW + LC)}{RW + RC + LW + LC} \times 100$$

UW $\geq 25\%$ **Abnormal** (Barber & Stockwell, 1980)

(A **plus** sign indicates **UW to the left**, and a **minus** sign indicates **UW to the right**.)

Bilateral Weakness

When the total strength of the caloric responses (denominator) is less than 30 degrees/sec, it can be defined as **bilateral weakness** (Barber & Stockwell, 1980). **BW** is usually an indication of both peripheral and central abnormality.

In case of bilateral weakness, an ice-water irrigation can possibly be used to determine any functionality of the peripheral vestibular organs.

Caloric - Both Eyes

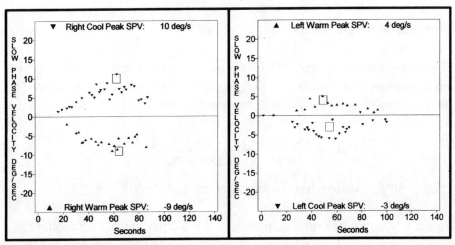

Caloric Weakness: 46% in the left ear

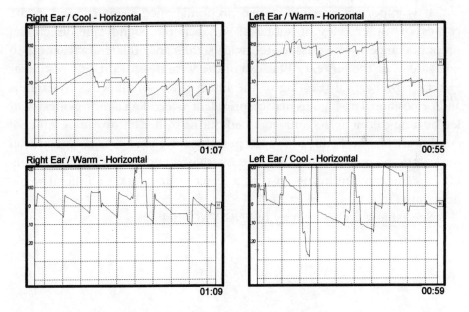

Figure 28. Significant unilateral weakness (46%) to the left side. "Pods" shape (*top*) for the left ear is shallow as compared to the "rounded liplike" shape for the right ear, depicting asymmetry of caloric responses.

Directional Preponderance

Directional preponderance compares the strengths between the right-beating nystagmus (RW and LC conditions) and the left-beating nystagmus (LW and RC conditions). The formula to calculate DP is:

$$DP = \frac{(RW + LC) - (LW + RC)}{RW + LC + LW + RC} \times 100$$

DP >30%   Abnormal (Barber & Stockwell, 1980)

Unlike UW, a plus or minus sign in the calculation does not mean any localized abnormality. A significant DP is nonlocalizing, however, and is an abnormal indication of peripheral and/or central disorders.

It is important that directional preponderance is interpreted in the context of other relevant subtests. For example, significant directional preponderance is often associated with significant unilateral weakness to one side (e.g., the left ear). Because of the weakness of the left vestibular system, right-beating (beating to the intact side) spontaneous nystagmus and/or positional nystagmus may be prevalent, overriding almost nonexistent left-beating caloric nystagmus induced during either left-warm or left-cool conditions, obviously due to the left peripheral weakness. Consequently, all the caloric responses could become overwhelmingly right-beating, resulting in significant DP, in this case, as a result of unilateral peripheral weakness in the left.

See Table 4 for a summary of ENG/VNG findings.

Summary of ENG/VNG Findings

Table 4. Summary of ENG/VNG findings with gross indications either peripheral or central in nature. These indications, of course, need to be interpreted in conjunction with the patient's case history and other clinical findings.

Subtests	Indications if Abnormal
Saccade	Central (PPRF)
Pursuit	Central
Gaze	Peripheral (Spontaneous nystagmus)
Positional	Peripheral (Positional nystagmus)
Optokinetic	Central
Dix-Hallpike	Peripheral (BPPV)
Caloric	Peripheral (Unilateral/bilateral weakness)

PPRF = paramedian pontine reticular formation; BPPV = benign paroxysmal positional vertigo.

Rotational Chair

(CPT Codes: 92546)

In addition to the caloric test, the vestibulo-ocular reflex (VOR) can also be examined by placing the patient in a chair in darkness during the **rotational chair** test, and the characteristics of the VOR can be recorded while the chair is rotated in each direction (left-to-right and right-to-left) at a known frequency. The phase, gain, and symmetry of the slow-phase compensatory eye movement are examined. When the patient is rotated to the right, an increase in neural discharge occurs in the right horizontal semicircular canal (R_{SCC}) while neural discharge decreases in the left SCC (L_{SCC}) (Fig. 29). The cupula deflection medially toward the ampulla in the rightward rotation is often referred to as an **ampullopetal pull** inside the R_{SCC}. In the L_{SCC}, an **ampullofugal pull** (away from ampulla) to the opposite direction produces a decrease in neural discharge. This neural difference between the right and left canals causes the eyes to deviate slowly toward the side of the weaker neural discharge (leftward in this case) or, in terms of physiologic mechanism, in the same direction as the horizontal SCC cupula deflection and endolymph flow. This **slow** compensatory deviation represents the **vestibular phase** of the nystagmus eye movement. The **fast** phase (saccade) of the eye movement is considered to be generated within the paramedian pontine reticular formation (PPRF), and "**beats**" in the same direction as the head is turning (i.e., right-beating nystagmus). Because of the bilateral response, each vestibular system cannot be tested independently. This test, therefore, is best combined with the caloric test to determine the relative strength of the horizontal semicircular canal.

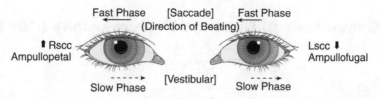

RIGHT BEATING NYSTAGMUS
(Rotating to the Right; RW; LC)

Fast Phase [Saccade] Fast Phase
(Direction of Beating)

↑ Rscc
Ampullopetal

Lscc ↓
Ampullofugal

[Vestibular]
Slow Phase Slow Phase

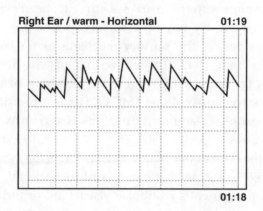

Right Ear / warm - Horizontal   01:19

01:18

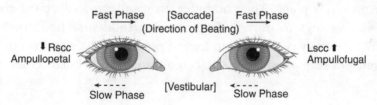

LEFT BEATING NYSTAGMUS
(Rotating to the Left; LW; RC)

Fast Phase [Saccade] Fast Phase
(Direction of Beating)

↓ Rscc
Ampullopetal

Lscc ↑
Ampullofugal

[Vestibular]
Slow Phase Slow Phase

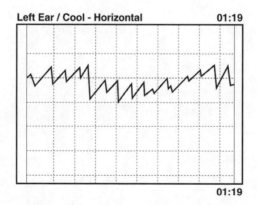

Left Ear / Cool - Horizontal   01:19

01:19

Figure 29. Principles of the VOR depicting the basic mechanism of generating right/left-beating nystagmus.

Computerized Dynamic Posturography (CDP)

(CPT Code: 92548)

While the VNG/ENG and rotational chair test battery examines the vestibular system in combination with the visual system (e.g., head-eye coordination), **dynamic posturography** attempts to incorporate the examination of proprioception as part of the sensory mechanisms for balance (Black & Nashner, 1985; Nashner, 1982, 1985a; 1985b). Thus, the dynamic posturography consists of two subtests known as the **sensory organization test (SOT)** and the **motor control test (MCT)**. The test protocol can be computerized (i.e., **computerized dynamic posturography**, **CDP**) to allow sophisticated analysis of postural integrity (Nashner, 1993).

In the SOT, the patient (suspended in a harness for safety) is placed on a "sway-referenced" platform that can record the patient's center of mass over time, while the patient's vestibular, visual, and proprioceptive inputs are altered systematically (e.g., present, absent, or distorted). The different profiles are generated to suggest vestibular, visual, and/or proprioceptive abnormality (Fig. 30).

In the MCT, the same platform moves unpredictably either in the anterior or posterior plane. The computer program can analyze the patient's correction strategy to prevent falling during sudden shifts in body mass (e.g., ankle strategy versus hip strategy to prevent a fall). Incorrect or abnormal strategies may possibly be corrected through vestibular rehabilitation.

SENSORY ORGANIZATION TEST (SOT)-SIX CONDITIONS

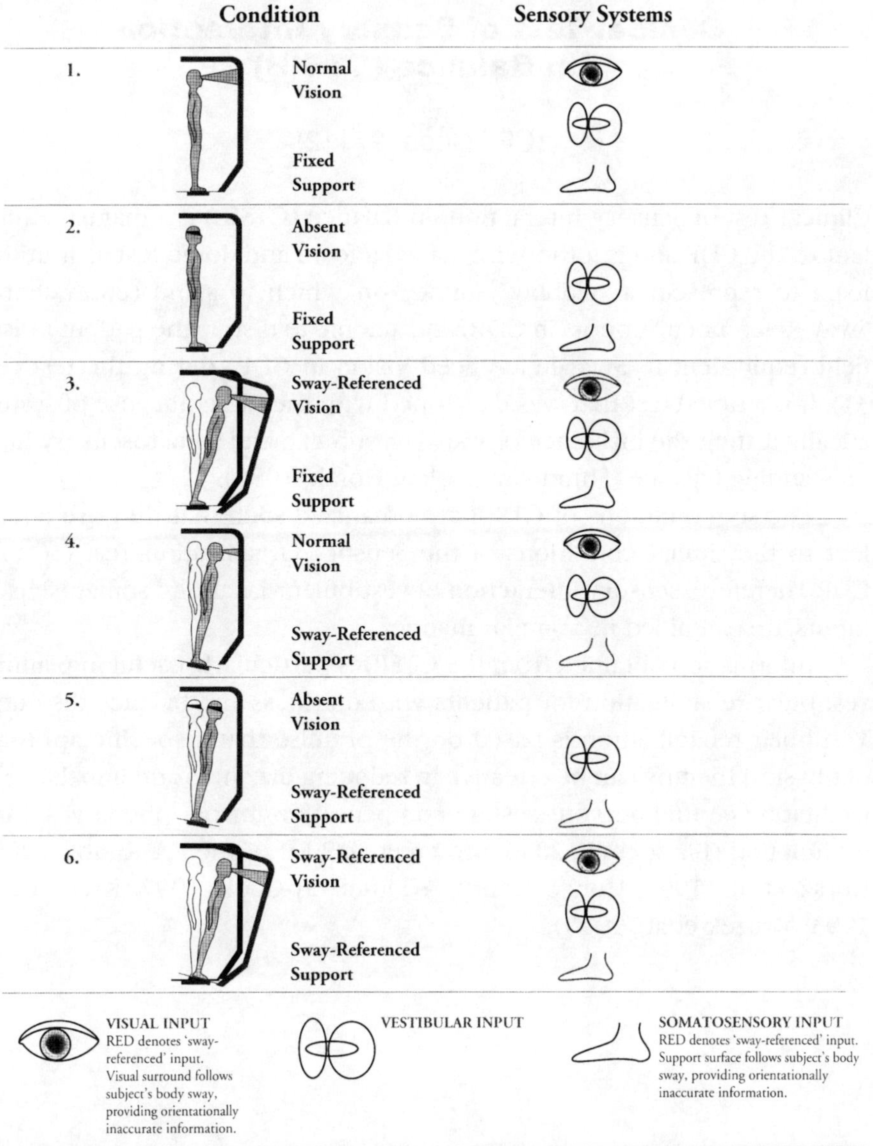

	Condition	Sensory Systems
1.	Normal Vision / Fixed Support	
2.	Absent Vision / Fixed Support	
3.	Sway-Referenced Vision / Fixed Support	
4.	Normal Vision / Sway-Referenced Support	
5.	Absent Vision / Sway-Referenced Support	
6.	Sway-Referenced Vision / Sway-Referenced Support	

VISUAL INPUT
RED denotes 'sway-referenced' input. Visual surround follows subject's body sway, providing orientationally inaccurate information.

VESTIBULAR INPUT

SOMATOSENSORY INPUT
RED denotes 'sway-referenced' input. Support surface follows subject's body sway, providing orientationally inaccurate information.

Figure 30. An organizational chart of six conditions of Sensory Organization Test (SOT) (Courtesy of NeuroCom International). Failure in conditions 5 and 6 in particular is a good indication for vestibular impairments.

Clinical Test of Sensory Interaction
on Balance (CTSIB)

(CPT Code: 97112)

Clinical Test of Sensory Interaction on Balance (CTSIB) is a manual equivalent to the CDP and is, otherwise, called a foam and dome test as it utilizes foam to represent a "wobbly" surface on which to stand (equivalent to Sway-Referenced Support in CDP) and a dome to distort the patient's visual field (equivalent to Sway-Referenced Vision in CDP) during the test (Fig. 31). It is a timed test that was developed with the same purpose of systematically testing the influence of visual, vestibular, and somatosensory input on standing balance (Shumway-Cook & Horak, 1986).

The six conditions of CTSIB are organized such that they are equivalent to the similar conditions of the Sensory Organization Test (SOT) in CDP. Therefore, sensory interaction of vestibular, visual, and somatosensory inputs are examined in a similar manner.

Information obtained from the CTSIB is particularly useful in planning vestibular rehabilitation for patients with dizziness and balance disorders. Vestibular rehabilitation is based on the premise that a specific approach of physical therapy can be effective in reducing dizziness and imbalance by facilitating central nervous system compensation for peripheral vestibular dysfunction (Black et al., 2000; Brown et al, 2001; Cohen & Kimball, 2003; Horak et al., 1992; Horak, Henry, & Shumway-Cook, 1997; Krebs et al., 1993; Mruzek et al., 1995).

Clinical Test of Sensory Interaction on Balance (CTSIB)
UHA Physician Office Center
Audiology – WVU Department of Otolaryngology
Morgantown, West Virginia
(304) 598-4825

The CTSIB is a timed test that was developed for systematically testing the influence of visual, vestibular, and somatosensory input on standing balance.

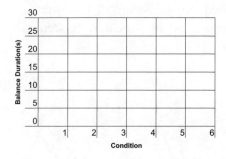

Conditions

1) Quiet standing on the floor, looking straight ahead.

2) Quiet standing on the floor, with eyes closed.

3) Quiet standing on the floor, wearing the conflict dome.

4) Quiet standing on the foam, with eyes open.

5) Quiet standing on the foam, with eyes closed.

6) Quiet standing on the foam, wearing the conflict dome.

Procedures
Patients can be tested in a quiet, well-lighted room with a linoleum floor. Position yourself to be able to support the patient in case of a fall.

Each patient is instructed to **"stand quietly with your feet together, hands across your waist, and look straight ahead as long as possible. Do this until I tell you to stop."** Include the instruction to **"close your eyes"** for condition 2 and **"Now, I'd like you to wear this hat and look at the cross"** for condition 3. Patients are asked to stand **"on the center of the foam"** for conditions 4 through 6.

Perform two trials for each condition. Each trial would last for up to 30 seconds. Use a stopwatch. Record in the bar graph above how long each trial lasted in each condition. A trial should be terminated when the patient's arms or feet change position. Rest the patient between trials, for 30 to 60 seconds, to eliminate the confounding affect of fatigue. The entire test should take no more than 20 minutes.

Interpretation
Condition 1 – Reference
Condition 2 – Examines how well patients maintain balance in the absence of any vision.
Condition 3 – Examines how well patients maintain balance when vision is present but that information conflicts with vestibular information.
Condition 4,5, and 6 – Involve standing on foam and repeating the visual conditions described for Conditions 1 through 3.

Test Results	Possible Diagnosis
Abnormal 3	Abnormal reliance on vision for postural control. (e.g. Post-concussion Vest. Syndrome, BPPV)
Abnormal 3-6	Sensory interaction problem.
Abnormal 5-6	Vestibular Impairments

Clinical Impression

Figure 31. Clinical Test of Sensory Interaction on Balance. (Reproduced with permission from Shumway-Cook & Horak, 1986.) (Adapted from Shumway-Cook, A. & Horak, F. [1986]. The influence of sensory interaction of balance: Suggestion from the field, *Physical Therapy, 65*, 1548–1550, with permission of the American Physical Therapy Association. This material is copyrighted, and any further reproduction or distribution is prohibited.)

Vestibular Rehabilitation

A vestibular rehabilitation program for dizzy patients is based on the premise that the central nervous system (CNS) compensation of vestibular disease/weakness can be facilitated through use of repeated "systematic" exercises (Figs. 32 and 33).

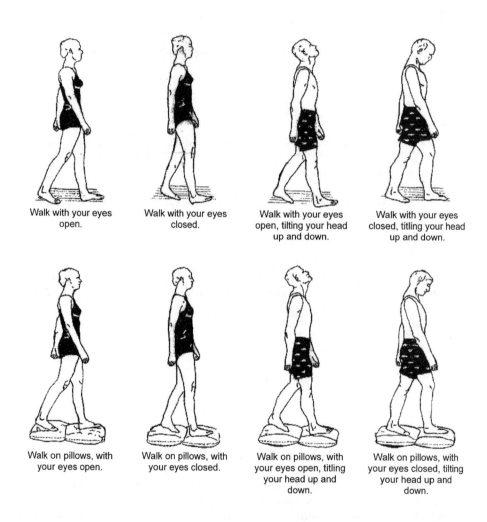

Figure 32. Various walking exercises on two different surfaces with either eyes open or closed while a patient moves the head up and down (adapted from Hamid, 1997).

Repeat the following sequence of exercises three times a day. Each exercise should be done 10-15 times during the sequence. Continue with these exercises for 2-3 months.

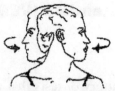

While seated, with eyes open, turn your head from side to side. First slowly, and then gradually increase speed according to your own pace.

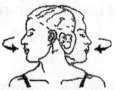

While seated, with your eyes closed, turn your head from side to side. First slowly, and then gradually increase speed according to your own pace.

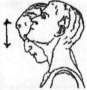

While seated, with eyes open, move your head up and down. Slowly and then gradually increase speed at your own pace.

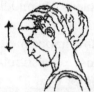

While seated, with eyes closed, move your head up and down. Slowly and then gradually increase speed at your own pace.

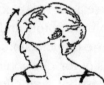

While seated, with eyes open, turn your head to the right 45 degrees. Shake your head up and down.

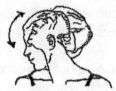

While seated, with eyes closed, turn your head to the right 45 degrees. Shake your head up and down.

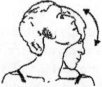

While seated, with eyes open, turn your head to the left 45 degrees. Shake your head up and down.

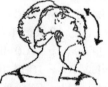

While seated, with eyes closed, turn your head to the left 45 degrees. Shake your head up and down.

Figure 33. Various head movement exercises with either eyes open or closed while a patient is sitting down upright (adapted from Hamid, 1997).

Vestibular-Evoked Myogenic Potentials (VEMP)

(CPT Code: 92585)

The VEMP is a relatively recent addition to a battery of tests that are used in the diagnosis of superior canal dehiscence (SCD) syndrome (Minor, 2000; Streubel et al., 2001) and other vestibular-related disorders (Zhou & Cox, 2004). Patients with SCD syndrome present with vertigo and nystagmus induced by loud noises (Tullio phenomenon) as well as by stimuli that result in changes in middle ear or intracranial pressure. It has been reported that the dehiscence of bone overlying the superior semicircular canal creates a low-impedance pathway ("third mobile window") that increases the response of vestibular and auditory receptors to sound and pressure stimuli (Minor et al., 1998). It is noteworthy that some patients with SCD present with either unilateral or bilateral conductive hearing loss.

VEMP responses are considered to be of vestibular origin (more specifically, inferior vestibular nerve) (Murofushi et al., 1996) and can be elicited by clicks and recorded in a manner similar to ABR, although the placement of the electrodes is slightly different (e.g., active electrode on the sternocleidomastoid muscle halfway between the mastoid and the clavicle; reference electrode on the medial third of the clavicle along its anterior border; ground on the sternum). The intensity for clicks required to elicit a VEMP response in patients with normal vestibular function is typically greater than 85 dB nHL, even as loud as 100 dB nHL, whereas patients with SCD syndrome have been reported to have abnormally low thresholds for VEMP responses, as low as 70 dB nHL (Streubel et al., 2001) (Fig. 34). An alternative way to analyze the asymmetry of VEMP responses has recently been proposed (Akin & Murnane, 2001) in that side-to-side differences in terms of peak-to-peak amplitudes (A_L and A_R) elicited at a single intensity level (e.g., 100 dB nHL) are expressed as an asymmetry ratio (AR) calculated as: $AR = 100 \times [(A_L - A_R) / (A_L + A_R)]$; abnormal if AR >30 to 47%. Whichever analysis method you use, the VEMP results should be interpreted in combination with the characteristic symptoms, signs, and high resolution CT in the diagnosis of SCD.

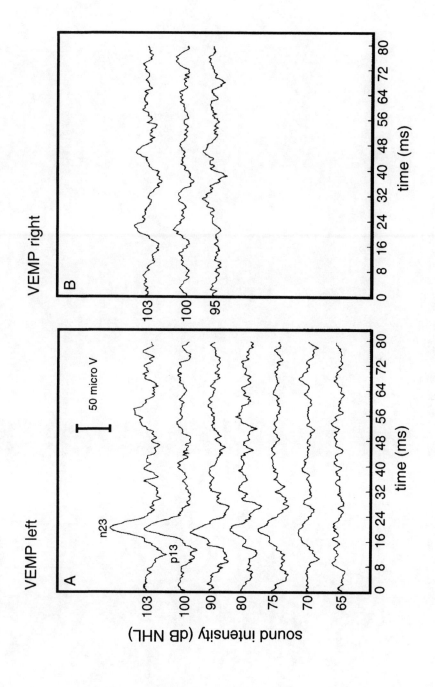

Figure 34. VEMP tracings (Streubel et al., 2001) from the normal side (*right*) where the VEMP is present at 100 dB nHL but disappears at 95 dB nHL, whereas the VEMP on the abnormal side (*left*) is present down to 70 dB nHL, significantly lower than the normal side.

PART III

Rehabilitation of Hearing Disorders

Once the degree and nature of hearing loss are diagnosed, habilitation and rehabilitation of hearing disorders must begin. This is primarily for the correction of improper speech and language in infants and children as hearing loss greater than a moderate degree is a major cause of speech and language delay in this population. Concerned parents can be advised to examine a checklist (see facing page) for the milestones of normal speech and language compiled by the National Institute on Deafness and Other Communication Disorders (NIDCD, 2005). If the hearing loss is identified at birth (e.g., **congenital**) or during early infancy due to either **progressive** (e.g., CMV) or **acquired** etiologies (e.g., bacterial meningitis), the intervention process is often referred to as "**habilitation**" as training must begin prior to acquisition of normal speech and language (i.e., **prelingual**) and actually involves the development of appropriate speech and language. On the other hand, the term "**rehabilitation**" refers to intervention after acquisition of normal speech and language (i.e., **postlingual**).

Technology such as hearing aids and cochlear implants may be sufficient for rehabilitation of the postlingual hearing loss, whereas the prelingual hearing loss requires extensive habilitation/rehabilitation.

Listed on the facing page is a checklist (NIDCD, 2005) that parents can follow to determine if their child's speech and language skills are developing on schedule. They should talk to their child's doctor about anything that is checked "no."

How Do I Know If My Child Is Reaching the Milestones?

	Yes	No
Birth to 5 months		
Reacts to loud sounds.	☐	☐
Turns head toward a sound source.	☐	☐
Watches your face when you speak.	☐	☐
Vocalizes pleasure and displeasure sounds (laughs, giggles, cries, or fusses).	☐	☐
Makes noise when talked to.	☐	☐
6 to 11 months		
Understands "no-no."	☐	☐
Babbles (says "ba-ba-ba" or "ma-ma-ma").	☐	☐
Tries to communicate by actions or gestures.	☐	☐
Tries to repeat your sounds.	☐	☐
12 to 17 months		
Attends to a book or toy for about two minutes.	☐	☐
Follows simple directions accompanied by gestures.	☐	☐
Answers simple directions nonverbally.	☐	☐
Points to objects, pictures, and family members.	☐	☐
Says two to three words to label a person or object (pronunciation may not be clear).	☐	☐
Tries to imitate simple words.	☐	☐
18 to 23 months		
Enjoys being read to.	☐	☐
Follow simple commands without gestures.	☐	☐
Points to simple body pasts such as "nose."	☐	☐
Understands simple verbs such as "eat," "sleep."	☐	☐
Correctly pronounces most vowels and *n, m, p, h,* especially in the beginning of syllables and short words. Also begins to use other speech sounds.	☐	☐
Says 8 to 10 words (pronunciation may still be unclear).	☐	☐
Asks for common foods by name.	☐	☐
Makes animal sounds such as "moo."	☐	☐
Starting combine words such as "more milk."	☐	☐
Begins to use pronouns such as "mine."	☐	☐

Hearing Aid Evaluation (HAE)

(CPT Codes: Monaural, 92590; Binaural, 92591)

A hearing aid is a miniature amplifier and has three main components:

1. **Microphone**: Picks up sounds and transforms acoustic energy to electric energy
2. **Amplifier**: Amplifies the sound
3. **Receiver**: Transforms the amplified electric energy to the louder acoustic energy

Other common components are: **volume control** to adjust the loudness, **telecoil** switch to get a better pickup with a telephone, **on/off switch**, and **batteries** as the source of power. Many modern digital hearing aids, however, have "automated" these options (with the exception of batteries).

Newer hearing aid technology has a **digital processing circuit** to process input signals clearly with less distortion and less internal noise. Digital technology is analogous to having a CD or DVD player as compared to an analog tape recorder or VHS video player. The distinctive features of digital processing may include speech enhancement in noisy environments, placing optimal speech signals within the hearing-impaired patient's narrow dynamic range, feedback cancellation, and frequency modification to fit the patient's hearing loss (Fig. 35).

SPEECH PROCESSING THROUGH HEARING AID

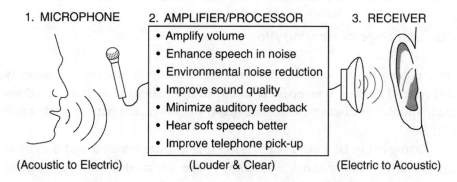

1. MICROPHONE

(Acoustic to Electric)

2. AMPLIFIER/PROCESSOR

- Amplify volume
- Enhance speech in noise
- Environmental noise reduction
- Improve sound quality
- Minimize auditory feedback
- Hear soft speech better
- Improve telephone pick-up

(Louder & Clear)

3. RECEIVER

(Electric to Acoustic)

MINIATURIZATION
(And, yes, it still needs a battery)

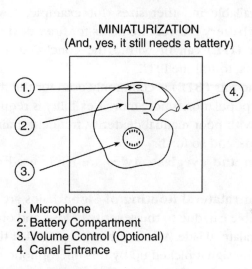

1. Microphone
2. Battery Compartment
3. Volume Control (Optional)
4. Canal Entrance

Figure 35. Typical electroacoustic components of a hearing aid. Most hearing aids commercially sold today are "digitally" processed, thus accomplishing not only amplification (making sounds louder) but also speech processing (enhanced speech clarity especially in noise, noise reduction, reducing auditory feedback, etc.).

Size and Style of Hearing Aids

Different styles of hearing aids are available depending on the severity and type of hearing loss, specific needs of the patient (e.g., complications from middle ear diseases, anatomic malformations), and patient preference (Fig. 36).

Completely-In-Canal (CIC) is the smallest size available and the entire aid fits inside the ear canal. Patients who are "cosmetically" conscientious typically prefer the CIC, but they must be counseled as to restricted features that may be available in other sizes, for example, fewer programming options, shorter battery life, requirements for finer dexterity.

In-The-Ear (ITE) can fit within the concha area, and varies from canal, half-concha, to full-shell ITE.

Behind-The-Ear (BTE) is commonly used for the more severe losses or the pediatric population where more flexibility is required. It is also useful for patients with poor manual dexterity, frequent drainage from middle ear complications, and so forth.

Body-worn and eyeglass styles are rarely used in today's clinical practice.

CROS (Contralateral Routing of Signal) aids are used for patients with one unaidable ear, due to the severity of loss, and one normal hearing ear on the contralateral side. A microphone is placed at the ear level of the "bad" side and the signal picked up by this microphone is "routed" (either through a hard-wire or an FM transmitter) to the receiver in the ear level hearing aid on the "good" or normal ear. If the better ear also has a hearing loss, the arrangement is called **BICROS**, indicating that a microphone and an amplifier are also placed on the side of the better ear.

BAHA (Bone-Anchored Hearing Aid) as part of advanced technology should also be considered as an alternative option to a traditional CROSS hearing aid for patients with profound unilateral hearing loss and, of course, patients with bilateral atresia.

CIC	CANAL	HALF CONCHA	FULL CUSTOM	MINI and POWER BTE'S

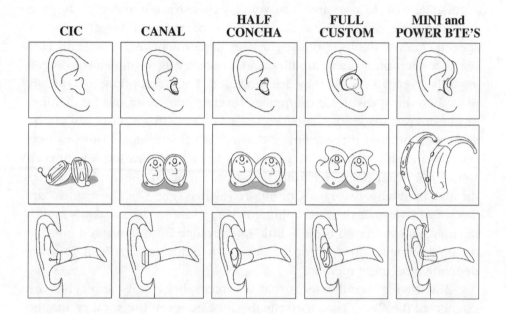

Figure 36. Lateral and cross-sectional views of various hearing aids in different sizes, for example, Completely-in-Canal (CIC), Canal, Half Concha, Full Custom, Behind-the-Ear (BTE) models (based on a display from Widex Hearing Aid Company). Prices vary according to size with a smaller size being more expensive.

Assistive Listening Devices

Assistive listening devices (ALDs) are resources that could help the hard of hearing to communicate more easily. The devices are often readily accessible, easy to use, and relatively inexpensive compared to hearing aids. The main goal of these devices is to "bring in the target sound or speech closer to the listener with hearing impairment." ALDs typically consist of a microphone, an amplifier, and a receiver as in miniaturized hearing aids, except in ALDs they are separated. The microphone is typically placed on the speaker, for example, a teacher in a classroom for children or in front of a television's speaker. The receiver with amplifier is worn by a hearing-impaired listener either through small earplugs, foam headsets (like a Walkman), or booted directly into the patient's hearing aids. Speech sounds are then delivered from the microphone to the receiver either through hard-wire, FM signals, or infrared signals (Fig. 37). The main advantage of ALDs is that the microphone is very close to the speaker's mouth or the sound source so there is little interference from unwanted noise in the environment. The cost for the device, its utility, and its flexibility vary depending on these methods.

Hard-wire literally means that the microphone and the receiver are connected through a cord with the distance between the speaker and the listener being restricted by the length of the cord, for example, 10 to 15 feet. Obviously, mobility would be restricted and somewhat cumbersome, but it is most economical.

FM does not require any wire, thus mobility is greatly enhanced. The signals can be easily transmitted within a typical classroom, living room, or even in a large auditorium such as a concert hall or a church.

Infrared is very similar to the FM except that the signals are transmitted by infrared light. Thus, one of the disadvantages for infrared is interference from sunlight. You should avoid, therefore, purchasing the infrared device if you intend to use it in a bright living room where sunlight shines in freely.

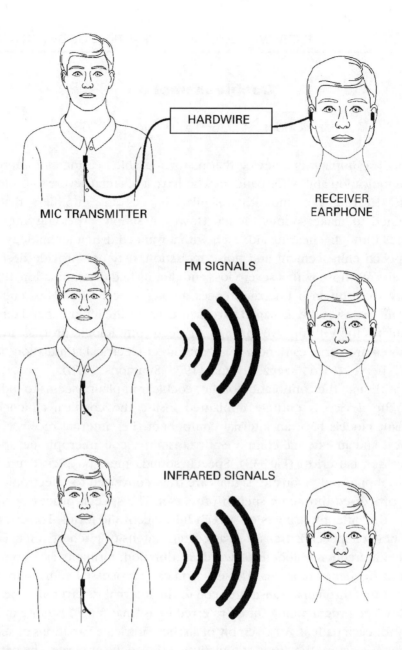

HARDWIRE

MIC TRANSMITTER

RECEIVER
EARPHONE

FM SIGNALS

INFRARED SIGNALS

Figure 37. Schematic drawing of three different ALD methods, namely, hardwire, FM, infrared. The main purpose of all these devices is to enhance so-called "signal-to-noise ratio" (S/N) by placing a microphone right at the speaker's mouth and a receiver (e.g., ear piece) at a listener's ears.

Cochlear Implant

(CPT Codes: 92626, 92601 through 92604)

A cochlear implant is a device that restores usable hearing and improved communication ability for patients who have a bilateral severe-to-profound SNHL. Hearing aids and other similar devices are amplifiers that are designed to make sounds louder. However, simply providing amplified sounds through a hearing aid, even with advanced digital technology such as speech enhancement and noise reduction, may not provide desirable benefits for those with a severe loss and diminished discrimination, that is, ability to distinguish fine differences among speech sounds. A cochlear implant bypasses the damaged part (hair cells) of the inner ear and directly stimulates the VIIIth nerve through an electrophysiologic process. In fact, early research articles denote it as "the direct electrical stimulation of the VIIIth nerve" (Clark, Kranz, & Minas, 1973; Simmons, 1979).

Although the connotation of the "cochlear implant " seems to indicate that the device is entirely implanted inside the cochlea, all cochlear implant models have an internal component (i.e., internal receiver, electrodes) and an external component (transmitter coil, microphone, speech processor, batteries) (Fig. 38). Speech sounds must be picked up by a microphone, and "acoustic" signals are then converted to "electronic" signals processed through a speech processor. The speech processor "translates" the different aspects of speech into electronic forms. For example, loudness of speech is translated as current intensity, pitch of voice as fundamental frequency, length of words as duration, formants as a combination of frequency domains. The electronically processed sounds are then transmitted through a transmitter coil to the internal receiver and the electrodes. The programming (often referred to as "mapping") is done individually for each patient. An assembly of all these intricate variations of speech becomes a part of the direct stimulation of the cochlear nerve. The patients describe those processed sounds as much like a robot talking with a mechanical-sound quality. They will need to go through an extensive rehabilitation process.

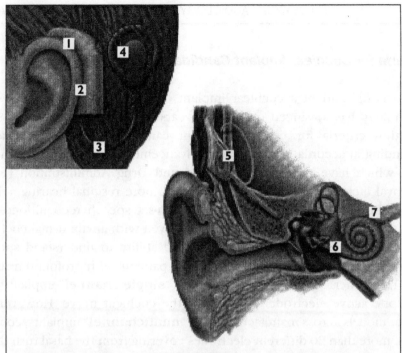

The Nucleus cochlear implant system works in the following manner:

1. Sounds are picked up by the small, directional microphone located in the ear level processor.

2. The speech processor filters, analyzes and digitizes the sound into coded signals.

3. The coded signals are sent from the speech processor to the transmitting coil.

4. The transmitting coil sends the coded signals as FM radio signals to the cochlear implant under the skin.

5. The cochlear implant delivers the appropriate electrical energy to the array of electrodes, which has been inserted into the cochlea.

6. The electrodes along the array stimulate the remaining auditory nerve fibers in the cochlea.

7. The resulting electrical sound information is sent through the auditory system to the brain for interpretation.

Pictures courtesy of Cochlear Ltd.

Figure 38. Assembly of external (1–4) and internal (5–7) components of the Nucleus cochlear implant system by Cochlear Americas Ltd.

Criteria for Cochlear Implant Candidacy

When is the patient a cochlear implant candidate? As cochlear implant technology has advanced over many years of clinical trials since 1985, selection criteria for cochlear implant candidacy have been steadily expanding in accordance with these advancements. Current selection criteria which have met necessary Food and Drug Administration (FDA) approval include: Adults and children with more residual hearing; adults and children with more preoperative open-set speech recognition; children as young as 12 months; and persons even with an abnormal cochlea.

Research has demonstrated improved ability to understand speech through the cochlear implant even among patients with profound hearing loss. The earlier clinical trial began with a "**single channel**" implant with only one active electrode to stimulate the cochlear nerve. However, all recent models across manufacturers are "**multichannel**" implants, consisting of more than 20 different electrodes covering from the basal turn (high frequency) to the apical turn (low frequency) of the cochlea. Incorporating the "**place theory of hearing**," where coding of frequency information depends on the place along the basilar membrane, the multichannel implants seem to provide much better speech understanding than the single-channel implants. All implant manufacturers also provide an ear level external device for adults and children while offering a body-worn speech processor for infants as an alternative.

2004 Candidacy for Cochlear Implant Criteria*

Minimum age	Adults and Children (above 12 mo)
Onset of hearing loss	Pre and Postlingual
Degree of hearing loss	Profound (below 2 years of age) Severe to profound (above 2 years)
Speech recognition	Adults: 50% or less on open-set sentence recognition in the ear to be implanted and 60% or less in nonimplanted ear or binaurally; receive little or no benefit from hearing aids Children: Lack of progress in auditory skills; receive little or no benefit from hearing aids
Medical contraindications	Contraindications to surgery; Deformity of the ear such as Mondini must be weighted in risks/benefits consideration
Developmental factors	Other developmental disorders must be weighted in terms of risks/benefits
Motivation and expectations	High motivation and appropriate expectations from both patient and family

*According to Cochlear Nucleus 24 Model

Success Hierarchy from Cochlear Implant

The degree of success with cochlear implant varies depending on how one defines "success." Most patients seeking an option of cochlear implant expect that they or their children will, in time, be able to communicate through listening and speaking. Because successful outcomes also depend on many variables and are very different from patient to patient, the following success hierarchy was proposed according to three main categories of these variables: onset of profound bilateral deafness, duration of auditory deprivation, and type of educational training (Northern et al., 1986). Deafness can be present at birth (**congenital**) or **acquired** during infancy (e.g., meningitis). Children with acquired hearing loss who have had even a few years of exposure to the speech and language process through normal hearing tend to do better than children with congenital hearing loss. However, this variable can be confounded by duration of auditory deprivation. Infants with congenital deafness whose hearing loss is **identified early** through early hearing screening (Yoshinaga-Itano et al., 1998) can be implanted at a minimum age of 12 months, making duration of auditory deprivation minimal. Patients with acquired hearing loss, but with a long period of auditory deprivation, have a poorer prognosis for success. Type of educational training must also be taken into consideration in addition to the desire of patients and/or their parents with respect to communication methodology. The more auditory input that is included in the training, the better the success with oral (speaking) communication through audition (listening) seems to be expected. Inclusion of proper language development with any method also seems to play a key role in overall language development (Yoshinaga-Itano et al., 1998). Factors such as family support, motivation, and involvement of other mental and/or developmental disorders play a role in determining the outcome. The answer probably lies along a continuum of success probability (Table 5), and potential candidates and their family members must be counseled accordingly.

Continuum of Success Probability

Table 5. Possible Success Hierarchy from Cochlear Implant.

	Low	High
Onset	Congenital	Acquired
Identification	Late	Early
Auditory Deprivation	Long-term	Short-term
Training Method	Less Auditory	More Auditory
Use of Speech	Less Oral	More Oral
Language	Less Language	More Language
Family Support	Less	More
Motivation	Low	High
Other Disorders	Yes	None

Modified from Northern et al. (1986).

Methods of Rehabilitation

(CPT Codes: 92626 and 92627)

There are numerous methods of habilitation/rehabilitation for hearing-impaired patients (Table 6). The appropriateness of a certain methodology depends on the degree and nature of loss, age of onset, existence of other developmental disorders, and philosophy of patients or their parents with regard to intervention. It should be emphasized that an ultimate decision as to choice of the method rests on patients or their parents as such decision encompass not only the factors associated with hearing loss but also social and even religious issues surrounding the impairment. Professionals in health care and education should take an "advisory" role in such decision-making processes.

In general, the methodologies can be organized into three categories: **total communication**, **oral methods**, and **auditory methods**. *Total communication* refers to intervention where manual sign language, lipreading and auditory input are all integrated into the development of speech and language. It is commonly used for prelingual children with severe-to-profound sensorineural hearing loss. *Oral methods* extensively incorporate the use of lipreading and other visual cues in the correction of speech errors. *Auditory methods* emphasize the use of audition as the primary mode of sensory input, although the extent of how it limits the use of other sensory cues may differ across various auditory methodologies. The **auditory-verbal method** (Pollack, 1970), for example, restricts any other sensory cues except audition during training. The **cued speech method** (Cornett, 1972) organizes uniquely developed "cues" to help in detecting certain features of speech sounds that are difficult for the hearing-impaired to recognize as some speech sounds possess identical lipreading features (e.g., voiced /b/ vs. voiceless /p/). A methodology such as the **Verbotonal method** (Asp, 2006; Guberina, 1964, 1972) incorporates multisensory input such as visual, tactile, and even proprioceptive cues in speech and language remediation, although the ultimate goal is still to enable speech communication primarily through audition.

Summary of Rehabilitation Methods

Table 6. Summary of Various Habilitation/Rehabilitation Methods According to Use of Sign Language, Lipreading, Tactile Cues, Audition, and Speaking.

Type of Training	Sign	Lipreading	Tactile	Audition	Speaking
TC	Yes	Yes	Yes	Yes	Min
Oral	No	Yes	No	Yes	Yes
Cued	No	Yes	No	Yes	Yes
A-V	No	No	No	Yes	Yes
VT	No	Yes	Yes	Yes	Yes

Note: TC = Total Communication; Cued = Cued Speech; A-V = Auditory-Verbal; VT = Verbotonal

CONCLUSION

Proper treatment of acute and chronic hearing loss and/or balance disorders follows accurate diagnosis of those disorders. By working closely together, the physician and audiologist can provide appropriate and timely diagnostic, treatment, or rehabilitation options for the patient with hearing loss and/or balance disorders. Early detection of hearing loss is critical for minimizing the long-term effects of hearing loss; thus, consultation with an audiologist is recommended as soon as a possible hearing loss is suspected. A summary of common acute and chronic diseases that indicate physical and audiologic examinations is provided in Table 7.

Audiologic Tests for Common Ear Diseases

Table 7. Common Indications Associated with Frequently Used Audiologic and Vestibular Tests.

Indications	Otoscopy	Tympanometry	Audiometry	OAE	ABR	ECoG	VNG
ETD	Retracted	C	CHL	NL?	—	—	—
OM	Fluid	Bnv	CHL	Abn	—	—	—
BVT	Tubes	Blv	NL	NL?	—	—	—
ME Path	Abn	Abn	CHL	Abn	—	—	—
Otosclerosis	NL	A	CHL	Abn	—	—	—
Ménière's	NL	A	SNHL	Abn	NL	Abn	?
Retrocochlear	NL	A	SNHL	?	Abn	—	?

Note: ETD, eustachian tube dysfunction; OM, otitis media; BVT, bilateral ventilation tube; ME Path, middle ear pathology; OAE, otoacoustic emission; ABR, auditory brainstem response; ECoG, electrocochleography; VNG, videonystagmography; NL, normal; Abn, Abnormal; A, Type A normal tymp; Bnv, Type B tymp with normal volume; Blv, Type B tymp with large volume; C, Type C negative tymp; CHL, conductive hearing loss; SNHL, sensorineural hearing loss).

PART IV

References and Notes

In addition to references to the text, relevant background and information that is more technical in nature are *briefly* provided with references if appropriate.

Akin, F. W., & Murnane, O. D. (2001). Vestibular evoked myogenic potentials: preliminary report. *Journal of the American Academy of Audiology*, *12*, 445–452.

Amedee, R. G. (1995). The effects of chronic otitis media with effusion on the measurement of transiently evoked otoacoustic emissions. *Laryngoscope*, *105*, 589–595.

American National Standard Specifications for Audiometers (ANSI33.6-1969). (1970). New York: American National Standards Institute.

During the calibration of the audiometer, the sound pressure level (SPL) is measured through a standard earphone TDH-50 with an earphone cushion (MX-41/AR) that is specifically placed with 400–500 grams force onto a standard NBS 9-A coupler to verify that the earphone produces the specified SPL. For example, 0 dB HL is equivalent (or **calibrated**) to 11 dB SPL at 500 Hz, 6.5 dB SPL at 1000 Hz, and 8.5 dB SPL at 2000 Hz.

American Speech-Language-Hearing Association. (1990). Guidelines for audiometric symbols. *Asha*, *32*, 25–30.

Asp, C. W. (2006). *Verbotonal speech treatment*. San Diego, CA: Plural Publishing.

Baloh, R. W., & Honrubia, V. (2001). *Clinical neurophysiology of the vestibular system*. New York, NY: Oxford University Press.

Barber, H. O., & Stockwell, C. W. (1980). *Manual of electronystagmography*. St. Louis, MO: C. V. Mosby.

Bauch, C. D., & Olsen, W. O. (1986). The effect of 2000 to 4000 Hz hearing sensitivity on ABR results. *Ear and Hearing*, 7, 314–317.

Bauch, C. D., & Olsen, W. O. (1987). Average 2000 to 4000 Hz heaing sensitivity and ABR results. *Ear and Hearing*, 8, 184.

The table below, reproduced with permission from *Ear and Hearing*, provides a probability of expected abnormality *solely* as a function of average "peripheral" hearing loss for 2000, 3000, and 4000 Hz. As the average hearing loss increased above 70 dB HL, the probability of abnormality exceeds more than 50%.

Table 8. ABR data and sample size as a function of average hearing loss (dB HL) for 2000, 3000, and 4000 Hz

dB HL	ABR Results		
	% Normal	% Abnormal	Sample size
0–19	97	3	291
20–29	90	10	88
30–39	87	13	104
40–49	82	18	112
50–59	72	28	116
60–69	63	37	120
70–79	41	59	49
80–89	26	74	19
90–99	14	86	7
100+	0	100	10

Bess, F. H. (1985). The minimally hearing-impaired child. *Ear and Hearing*, *6*, 43-47.

Black, F. O., Angel, C. R., Pesznecker, S. C., & Gianna, C. (2000). Outcome analysis of individualized vestibular rehabilitation protocols. *American Journal of Otology*, *21*, 543-551.

Black, F. O., & Nashner, L. M. (1985). Postural control in four classes of vestibular abnormalities. In M. Igarashi, & F. O. Black (Eds.), *Vestibular and visual control of postural and locomotor equilibrium*. Basel: S. Karger.

Black, K. L., Oyer, R. F., & Seyfried, D. N. (1991). A clinical comparison of Grason Stadler insert earphones and TDH-50P standard earphones. *Ear and Hearing*, *12*, 361-362.

Boege, P., & Janssen, T. (2002). Pure-tone threshold estimation from extrapolated distortion product otoacoustic emission I/O-functions in normal and cochlear hearing loss ears. *Journal of the Acoustical Society of America*, *111*, 1810-1818.

Brodel, M. (1946). *Three unpublished drawings of the anatomy of the human ear*. Philadelphia: W. B. Saunders.

Brown, K. E., Whitney, S. L., Wrisley, D. M., & Furman, J. M. (2001). Physical therapy outcomes for persons with bilateral vestibular loss. *Laryngoscope*, *111*, 1812-1817.

Clark, G. M., Kranz, H. G., & Minas, H. (1973). Behavioral thresholds in the cat to frequency-modulated sound and electrical stimulation of the auditory nerve. *Experimental Neurology*, *41*, 190-200.

Clark, J. G. (1981). Uses and abuses of hearing loss classification. *Asha*, *23*, 493-500.

Clemis, J. D., Ballard, W. J., & Killion, M. C. (1986). Clinical use of an insert earphone. *Annals of Otology, Rhinology, and Laryngology*, *95*, 520-524.

Coats, A. C. (1981). The summating potential and Meniere's disease. I. Summating potential amplitude in Meniere's and non-Meniere's ears. *Archives of Otolaryngology*, *107*, 199-208.

Coats, A. C. (1986). Electrocochleography: Recording techniques and clinical applications. In J. Ferraro (Ed.), Electrocochleography. *Seminars in Hearing*, 7, 247-266.

Cohen H. S., & Kimball, K. T. (2003). Increased independence and decreased vertigo after vestibular rehabilitation. *Otolaryngology–Head and Neck Surgery*, *128*, 60-70.

Cone-Wesson, B., Dowell, R. C., Tomlin, D., Rance, G., & Ming, W. J. (2002). The auditory steady-state response: Comparisons with the auditory brainstem response. *Journal of the American Academy of Audiology*, *13*, 173-187.

Cornett, R. (1972). *Cued speech parent training and follow-up program*. Washington, DC: Bureau of Education for Handicapped DHEW, 96.

Davis, H., & Hirsh, S.K. (1976). A slow brainstem response for low frequency audiometry. *Audiology*, *15*, 181-195.

Dobie, R. A., Wilson, M. J. (1995). Comparison of objective threshold estimation procedures for 40 Hz auditory evoked potentials. *Ear and Hearing*, *15*, 299-310.

Durrant, J. D., Ferraro, J. A., Folsom, R. C., Weber, B. A., & Wolf, K., E. (1988*). The short latency auditory-evoked potentials.* A tutorial paper by the Working Group on Auditory Evoked Potential Measurements of the Committee on Audiologic Evaluation. Rockville, MD: ASHA.

Galambos, R., Makeig, S., & Talmachoff, P. (1981). A 40-Hz auditory potential recorded from the human scalp. *Proceedings of the National Academy of Science USA, 78,* 2643-2647.

Givens, G. D., & Seidemann, M. F. (1979). A systematic investigation of measurement parameters of acoustic reflex adaptation. *Journal of Speech and Hearing Disorders, 44,* 534-542.

Goodman, A. (1965). Reference zero levels for pure tone audiometer. *Asha, 7,* 262-263.

Gorga, M. P., Johnson, T. A., Kaminski, J. R., Beauchaine, K. L., Garner, C. A., & Neely, S. T. (2006). Using a combination of click-and tone burst-evoked auditory brain stem response measurements to estimate pure tone thresholds. *Ear and Hearing, 27,* 60-74.

Gorga, M. P., Neely, S. T., Bergman, B., Beauchaine, K. L., Kaminski, J. R., Peters, J., & Jesteadt, W. (1993). Otoacoustic emissions from normal-hearing and hearing-impaired subjects: Distortion product responses. *Journal of the Acoustical Society of America, 93,* 2050-2060.

Gorga, M. P., Neely, S. T., Dorn, P. A., & Hoover, B. M. (2003). Further efforts to predict pure-tone thresholds from distortion product otoacoustic emission input/output functions. *Journal of the Acoustical Society of America, 113,* 3275-3284.

Gorga, M. P., Neely, S. T., Ohlrich, B., Hoover, B., Redner, J., & Peters, J. (1997). From laboratory to clinic: A large scale study of distortion product otoacoustic emissions in ears with normal hearing and ears with hearing loss. *Ear and Hearing, 18,* 440-455.

Gorga, M. P., Reiland, J. R., Beauchaine, K. L., Worthington, D. W., & Jesteadt, W. (1987). Auditory brain stem responses from graduates of an intensive care nursery: Normal patterns of response. *Journal of Speech and Hearing Research, 30,* 311-318.

Guberina, P. (1964). Verbotonal method and its applications to the rehabilitation of the deaf. *Proceedings of the International Congress on Educaion of the Deaf* (p. 964). Washington, DC: Government Printing Office.

Guberina, P. (1972). *Case studies in the use of restricted bands of frequencies in auditory rehabilitation of the deaf.* Zagreb: Institute of Phonetics, Faculty of Arts of the University of Zagreb.

Hall, J. W., III. (1979). Auditory brainstem frequency following responses to waveform envelope periodicity. *Science, 205,* 1297-1299.

Hall, J. W., III. (1992). *Handbook of auditory-evoked responses*. Boston, MA: Allyn & Bacon.

Table values below, reproduced with permission from Allyn and Bacon, are useful in interpretation of the ABR results from newborns.

Table 9. ABR Latency and Amplitude Values for 80 dB HL Click Intensity Level in Newborns

CA (N)	Latency (msec)				
	I	V	I–III	III–V	I–V
33–34 (38)					
Mean	1.78	7.05	2.86	2.41	5.27
SD	0.30	0.39	0.28	0.26	0.36
35–36 (150)					
Mean	1.78	7.02	2.84	2.39	5.24
SD	0.26	0.38	0.27	0.25	0.36
37–38 (158)					
Mean	1.74	6.94	2.80	2.34	5.17
SD	0.21	0.42	0.31	0.26	0.40
39–40 (111)					
Mean	1.72	6.82	2.70	2.38	5.09
SD	0.23	0.38	0.27	0.25	0.36
41–42 (74)					
Mean	1.69	6.69	2.74	2.24	5.00
SD	0.19	0.29	0.22	0.21	0.30
43–44 (35)					
Mean	1.65	6.53	2.65	2.21	4.88
SD	0.15	0.32	0.26	0.21	0.31

Note. Reported by Gorga et al. (1987). Measurement parameters: stimulus—click, 0.1 msec, 80 dB HL (110 dB peSPL), 13/sec, monaural, Beyer DT48 earphone; acquisition—filters, 100–3,000 Hz; amplification, 100,000; sweeps, 1,024; analysis time, 15 msec; electrodes, Cz-Mi. CA = conceptional age in weeks; N = number of infants.

Table 10. ABR Latency and Amplitude Values as a Function of Intensity Level in Newborns

CA (N)	Wave V latency (msec)			
	80 dB	60 dB	40 dB	20 dB
33–34 (38)				
Mean	7.05	7.62	8.48	9.72
SD	0.39	0.41	0.49	0.56
35–36 (150)				
Mean	7.02	7.58	8.42	9.61
SD	0.38	0.43	0.54	0.67
37–38 (158)				
Mean	6.94	7.45	8.29	9.57
SD	0.42	0.44	0.51	0.74
39–40 (111)				
Mean	6.82	7.30	8.11	9.36
SD	0.38	0.40	0.49	0.57
41–42 (74)				
Mean	6.69	7.20	8.08	9.31
SD	0.29	0.29	0.35	0.54
43–44 (35)				
Mean	6.53	7.08	7.94	9.16
SD	0.32	0.33	0.51	0.53

Note. Reported by Gorga et al. (1987). Measurement parameters: stimulus—click, 0.1 msec, 13/sec, monaural, Beyer DT48 earphone; acquisition—filters, 100–3000 Hz; amplification, 100,000; sweeps, 1,024; analysis time, 15 msec; electrodes, Cz-Mi. CA = conceptional age in weeks; N = number of infants.

Table values below, reproduced with permission from Delmar Thomson Learning, are useful in interpretation of the ABR results from adults.

Table 11. Adult Normative ABR Latency Data

ABR component	Latency statistic		
	Mean (msec)	SD	+2.5 SD
I	1.54	0.10	1.79
III	3.70	0.15	4.08
V	5.60	0.19	6.08
I-III	2.20	0.16	2.60
III-V	1.84	0.17	2.26
I-V	4.04	0.18	4.49

Note. Reported by Schwartz, Pratt, and Schwartz (1989). Subjects: 20 subjects; 10 male, 10 female; age range of 19 to 36 years (mean age of 26 years); hearing threshold level criteria not specified. Measurement parameters: stimulus—type, click; duration, 0.1 msec; data are for rarefaction and condensation polarity combined; transducer, Etymotic ER-3A (note: latency data in table are corrected by 0.9 msec for tube acoustic transmission delay); intensity level, 80 dB nHL (108 dB SPL); stimulus rate was not specified; repetitions, 2000–4000 Hz. acquisition—bandpass filters, 100–1500 Hz; notch filter not indicated; analysis time, 15 msec; electrodes, Cz–A1. *SD* = standard deviation.

Hamid, M. A. (1997). Vestibular and balance rehabilitation. In G. B. Hughes (Ed.), *Clinical otology*. New York, NY: Thieme Medical.

Harford, E. R. (1975). Tympanometry. In J. Jerger (Ed.), *Handbook of clinical impedance audiometry*. Dobbs Ferry, NY: American Electromedics.

Haskins, H. (1949). *A phonetically balanced test of speech discrimination for children*. Unpublished master's thesis. Evanston, IL: Northwestern University.

Hirsh, I. J, Davis, H, Silverman, S. R, Reynolds, E. G, Eldert, E., & Benson, R. W. (1952). Development of materials for speech audiometry. *Journal of Speech and Hearing Disorders*, 17, 321–337.

Hood, J. D. (1960). The principles and practice of bone-conduction audiometry: A review of the present position. *Laryngoscope*, 70, 1211–1228.

Hood, L. J. (1998). *Clinical applications of the auditory brainstem response*. San Diego, CA: Singular Publishing Group.

Horak, F. B., Henry, S. M., Shumway-Cook, A. (1997). Postural perturbations: New insights for treatment of balance disorders. *Physical Therapy*, 77, 517–533.

Horak, F. B., Jones-Rycewicz, C., Black, F. O., & Sumway-Cook, A. (1992). Effects of vestibular rehabilitation on dizziness and imbalance. *Otolaryngology–Head and Neck Surgery*, 106, 175–180.

Hudgins, C. V., Hawkins, J. E., Karlin, J. E., & Stevens, S. S. (1947). The development of recorded auditory tests for measuring hearing loss for speech. *Laryngology*, 57, 57–89.

Jacobson, G. P. & Calder, J. H. (1998). A screening version of the dizziness handicap inventory (DHI-S). *American Journal of Otology*, 19, 804–808.

Jacobson, G. P., & Newman, C. W. (1990). The development of the dizziness handicap inventory. *Archives of Otolaryngology–Head and Neck Surgery*, 116, 424–427.

Jacobson, G. P., Newman, C. W. Hunter, L., & Balzer, G. K. (1991). Balance function test correlates of the Dizziness Handicap Inventory. *Journal of the American Academy of Audiology, 2*, 253–260.

Jerger, J. F. (1975). Diagnostic use of impedance measures. In J. Jerger (Ed.), *Handbook of clinical impedance audiometry*. Dobbs Ferry, NY: American Electromedics.

Jerger, J. F., Jerger, S., & Mauldin, L. (1972). Studies in impedance audiometry: I. Normal and sensorineural ears. *Archives of Otolaryngology, 96*, 513–581.

Jewett, D.L., & Williston, J. S. (1971). Auditory evoked far fields averaged from the scalp of humans. *Brain, 4*, 681–696.

Kemp, D. T. (1978). Stimulated acoustic emissions from within the human auditory system. *Journal of the Acoustical Society of America, 64*, 1386–1391.

Kemp, D. T. (1997). Otoacoustic emission in perspective. In M. S. Robinette & T. J. Glattke (Eds.), *Otoacoustic emissions: clinical applications*. New York, NY: Thieme.

Kei, J., Allison-Levick, J., Dockray, J., Harrys, R., Kirkegard, C., Wong, J., Maurer, M., Hegarty, J., Young, J., & Tudehope, D. (2003). High-frequency (1000-Hz) tympanometry in normal neonates. *Journal of the American Academy of Audiology, 14*, 20–28.

Keith, R. W. (1986). *SCAN: A screening test for auditory processing disorders*. San Diego, CA: Harcourt Brace Jovanovich.

Kirk, K. I, Pisoni, D. B, & Osberger, M. J. (1995). Lexical effects on spoken word recognition by pediatric cochlear implant users. *Ear and Hearing, 16*, 470–481.

Koike, K. J., Hurst, M. K., & Wetmore, S. J. (1994). Correlation between the American Academy of Otolaryngology–Head and Neck Surgery five-minute hearing test and standard audiologic data. *Otolaryngology–Head and Neck Surgery, 111*, 625–632.

Koike, K. J., & Wetmore, S. J. (1999). Interactive effects of the middle ear pathology and the associated hearing loss on transient-evoked otoacoustic emission measures. *Otolaryngology–Head and Neck Surgery, 121*, 238–244.

The TEOAE pass rates as shown in the figure below (reprinted with permission from *Otolaryngology–Head and Neck Surgery*) were 84% for Type A normal tympanograms, 6% for Type B_{NV} (normal volume), 60% for Type B_{LV} (large volume, i.e., open tubes), and 72% for Type C negative tympanograms.

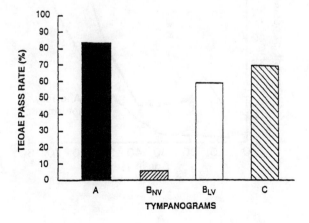

Krebs, D. E., Gill-Body. K. M., Riley, P. O., & Parker, S. W. (1993). Double-blind, placebo-controlled trial of rehabilitation for bilateral vestibular hypofunction: Preliminary report. *Otolaryngology–Head and Neck Surgery, 109,* 735–741.

Kummer, P., Janssen, T., & Arnold, W. (1998). The level and growth behavior of the 2 f1–f2 distortion product otoacoustic emission and its relationship to auditory sensitivity in normal hearing and cochlear hearing loss. *Journal of the Acoustical Society of America, 103,* 3431–3444.

Liden, G., & Kankkonen, A. (1961). Visual reinforcement audiometry. *Acta Otolaryngologica (Stockholm), 67,* 281–292.

Margolis, R. H., Bass-Ringdahl, S., Hanks, W. D., Holte, L., & Zapala, D. A. (2003). Tympanometry in newborn infants—1 kHz norms. *Journal of the American Academy of Audiology, 14,* 383–392.

Marshall, L., Heller, L. M., & Westhusin, L. J. (1997). Effect of negative middle-ear pressure on transient-evoked otoacoustic emissions. *Ear and Hearing, 18,* 218–226.

Martin, F. N. (1972). *Clinical audiometry and masking.* New York: Bobbs-Merrill.

Martin, F. N. (1985). The pseudohypacusic. In J. Katz (Ed.), *Handbook of clinical audiology.* Baltimore, MD: Williams & Wilkins.

Martin, F. N. (1986). *Introduction to audiology* (3rd ed.) Englewood Cliffs, NJ: Prentice-Hall.

Maurer, J. F., Rupp, R. R. (1979). *Hearing and aging.* New York, NY: Grune & Stratton.

Percentage of persons in the United States with auditory impairments at age 50 is about 20%, but rises to 30% at age 60, and to 50% at age 70. (Reproduced with permisionfrom Harris, C. S. *Fact book on aging: A profile of America's older population.* Washington, DC: National Council on the Aging, 1978, p. 100.)

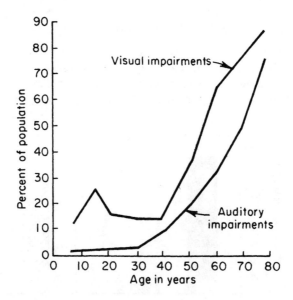

McKinley, A. M., Grose, J. H., & Roush, J. (1997). Multifrequency tympanometry and evoked otoacoustic emissions in neonates during the first 24 hours of life. *Journal of the American Academy of Audiology, 8,* 218–223.

Melnick, W. (1978). Temporary and permanent threshold shift. In D. M. Lipscomb (Ed.), *Noise and audiology.* Baltimore, MD: University Park.

Shown below is a pattern of hearing loss from typical industrial noise exposure as a function of frequency, reprinted with permission. The parameter is the number of years of working in the industrial noise environment. Data were adapted from Taylor, W., Pearson, J., Mair, A., & Burns, W. (1965). Study of noise and hearing in jute weaving. *Journal of the Acoustical Society of America, 38,* 113–1120.

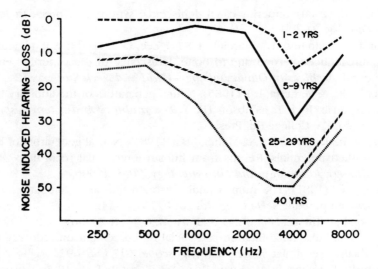

Metz, O. (1946). The acoustic impedance measured on normal and pathological ears. *Acta Otolaryngologica Supplement, 63,* 397–405.

Metz, O. (1952). Threshold of reflex contractions of muscles of middle ear and recruitment of loudness. *Archives of Otolaryngology, 55,* 536–543.

The Metz recruitment test demonstrated that the normal 70 to 95 dB Sensation Level (SL) required for elicitation of the acoustic reflex is markedly reduced (less than 60 dB) in ears with cochlear pathology.

Miller, M. H. (1986). *Occupational hearing conservation.* Austin, TX : Pro-Ed.

The first federal regulation to protect workers from harmful noise exposure was established as part of the Walsh-Harley Public Contracts in 1969. Since then, various regulations have been developed by the Occupational Safety and Health Administration (OSHA) to implement Occupational Hearing Conservation (OHC) programs. Once detailed noise analysis of the work environments is done, OSHA defines the *action level* for implementation of an OHC program as 85 dBA for a *time-weighted average (TWA)* of 8 hours, where the components of OHC program such as audiometric tests and administrative controls are required to be initiated. However, the actual permissible levels for workers are 90 dBA for an 8-hour TWA. Noise exposure is a trade-off between the intensity of noise measured in so-called A-weighted network (e.g., noted as dBA) to simulate the response characteristics (remember "equal loudness contour") of the human ear and duration of the exposure. So, if the worker is exposed to 95 dBA, a 5-dB higher level than 90 dBA, the duration of work must be reduced to half of 8 hours, that is, 4 hours, and at 100 dBA to only 2 hours. *Standard threshold shift (STS)* is defined as an average shift of 10 dB or more at 2000, 3000, and 4000 Hz relative to the baseline audiogram in either ear. OSHA requires that the employer inform the employee in writing that he or she has sustained a STS within 21 working days of the determination.

Minor, L. B. (2000). Superior canal dehiscence syndrome. *American Journal of Otology, 21,* 9–19.

Minor, L. B., Solomon, D., Zinreich, J. S., & Zee, D. S. (1998). Sound- and/or pressure-induced vertigo due to bone dehiscence of the superior semicircular canal. *Archives in Otolaryngology–Head and Neck Surgery, 124,* 249–258.

Moller, A. R., & Jannetta, P. J. (1985). Neural generators of the auditory brainstem response. In J. T. Jacobson (Ed.), *The auditory brainstem response.* San Diego, CA: College-Hill Press.

Moller, A. R., Jannetta, P. J., & Moller, M. B. (1981). Neural generators of brainstem evoked potentials: Results from human intercranial recordings. *Annals of Otology, Rhinology, and Lanryngology, 90,* 591–596.

Moore, J. K. (1987). The human auditory brainstem as a generator of auditory evoked potentials. *Hearing Research, 29,* 33–44.

Mruzek, M., Barin, K., Nichols, D. S., Burnett, C. N., & Welling, D. B. (1995). Effects of vestibular rehabilitation and social reinforcement on recovery following ablative vestibular surgery. *Laryngoscope, 105,* 686–692.

Murofushi, T., Halmagyi, M., Yavor, R. A., & Colebatch, J. G. (1996). Absent vestibular-evoked myogenic potentials in vestibular neurolabyrinthitis. *Archives of Otolaryngology–Head and Neck Surgery, 122,* 845–848.

Musiek, F. E. (1985). Application of central auditory test: An overview. In J. Katz (Ed.), *Handbook of clinical audiology.* Baltimore, MD: Williams & Wilkins.

Nashner, L. M. (1982). Adaptation of human movement to altered environments. *Trends in Neurosciences, 5,* 358–361.

Nashner, L. M. (1985a). Human movement control studies with the movable platform. In J. E. Desmedt (Ed.), *Motor control in man: Mechanism and clinical applications.* New York, NY: Raven Press.

Nashner, L. M. (1985b). Strategies for organization of human posture. In M. Igarashi, & F. O. Black (Eds.), *Vestibular and visual control of postural and locomotor equilibrium.* Basel: S. Karger.

Nashner, L. M. (1993). Computerized dynamic posturography. In G. P. Jacobson, C. W. Newman, & J. M. Kartush (Eds.). *Handbook of balance function testing.* Chicago, IL: Mosby–Yearbook.

National Institute on Deafness and Other Communication Disorders. (2005). Speech and language: Developmental Milestones. Available from: http://www.nidcd.nih.gov/health/voice/speechandlanguage.asp#mychild

Nilson, M., Soli, S. D., & Sullian, J. A. (1994). Development of the Hearing in Noise Test for the measurement of speech reception thresholds in quiet and in noise. *Journal of the Acoustical Society of America*, *95*, 1085–1099.

Northern, J. L. (1975). Clinical measurement procedures. In J. Jerger (Ed.), *Handbook of clinical impedance audiometry*. Dobbs Ferry, NY: American Electromedics.

Static compliance is a volume measurement of the middle ear cavity in terms of equivalent volume expressed in cubic centimeters (cc), although the actual measurement is done by measuring the sound pressure level (SPL) inside the ear canal and the value converted to the volume unit. The test takes two volume measurements. One volume (C_1, Physical Volume) is measured with the TM in a position of poor compliance, clamped at +200 mm/H_2O air pressure, where much of the sound (probe tone) is reflected against a stiffened TM, resulting in a higher SPL value in a smaller enclosed cavity. Thus, this measure is equivalent to the ear canal volume lateral to the TM (*top figure, below*, reprinted with permission from American Electromedics). Another volume (C_2, Equivalent Volume) is measured with the TM at maximum compliance, where sound is transmitted easily through the mobile TM, resulting in a maximum transmission of sound throughout the middle ear cavity and a lower SPL value due to a larger cavity encompassing the outer ear canal *and* middle ear cavity (*bottom figure, below*, reprinted with permission from American Electromedics). By subtracting the ear canal volume (C_1) from the combined volume of ear canal and middle ear cavity (C_2), the end product is the volume measure of the middle ear cavity, that is, the static compliance (C_3). Although the term "compliance" is used as part of the original classifications, it is the measure of the volume, not the compliance (mobility). The static compliance can vary depending on age, sex, and so forth (Jerger, Jerger, & Mauldin, 1972). In general, normal static compliance values range from between 0.3 cc and 1.6 cc.

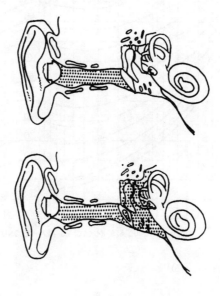

Northern, J. L., Black, F. O., Brimacombe, J. A., Cohen, N. L., Eisenberg, L. S., Kuprenas, S. V., Martinez, S. A., & Mischke, R. E. (1986). Selection of children for cochlear implantation. *Seminars in Hearing, 7,* 341–347.

Owens, J. J., McCoy, M. J., Lonsbury-Martin, B. L., & Martin, G. K. (1993). Otoacoustic emissions in children with normal ears, middle ear dysfunction, and ventilation tubes. *American Journal of Otology, 14,* 34–40.

Picton, T. W., Dimitrijevic, A., & John, M. S. (2002). Multiple auditory steady-state responses. *Annals of Otology, Rhinology, and Laryngology Supplement, 189,* 16–21.

Pollack, D. (1970). *Educational audiology for the limited-hearing infant.* Springfield, MA: Charles C Thomas.

Robertson, D. D., & Ireland, D. J. (1995). Dizziness Handicap Inventory correlates of computerized dynamic posturography. *Journal of Otolaryngology, 24,* 118–124.

Robinson, D. W., & Dadson, R. S. (1956). A re-determination of the equal loudness relations for pure tones. *British Journal of Applied Physics, 7,* 166–181.

Each contour below represents equal loudness as judged in units of *phons*. A phon is the sound pressure level (SPL) of a 1000-Hz reference tone that is judged to be equal in loudness to a test pure tone. For example, by definition, a 50-dB pure tone at 1000 Hz has a loudness of 50 phons. To be perceived as equally loud, the SPL of a 100–Hz tone must be raised to 60 dB (cross-point where the vertical axis at 100 Hz intersects the 50 phon contour), an increase of 10 dB over the 1000-Hz reference tone. (Figure reprinted with permission from the *British Journal of Applied Physics*.)

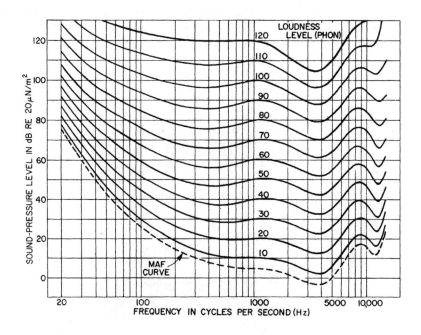

Roland, P. S., & Rutka, J. A. (2004). *Ototoxicity*. Hamilton, : BC Decker.

Schwartz, D. M., Pratt, R. E., Jr., & Schwartz, J. A. (1989). Auditory brainstem responses in preterm infants: Evidence of peripheral maturity. *Ear & Hearing, 10*, 14–22.

Shumway-Cook, A., & Horak, F. B. (1986). Assessing the influence of sensory interaction of balance: Suggestion from the field. *Physical Therapy, 66*, 1548–1550.

Simmons, B. F. (1979). Electrical stimulation of the auditory nerve in cats. Long-term electrophysiological and histological results. *Annals of Otology, Rhinology, and Laryngology, 88*, 533–539.

Streubel, S-O., Cremer, P. D., Carey, J. P., Weg, N., & Minor, L. B. (2001). Vestibular-evoked myogenic potentials in the diagnosis of superior canal dehiscence syndrome. *Acta Otolaryngologica Supplement, 545*, 41–49.

Suzuki, T., & Ogiba, Y. (1961). Conditioned orientation audiometry. *Archives of Otolaryngology, 74*, 192–198.

Tharpe, A. M., & Bess, F. H. (1999). Minimal, progressive, and fluctuating hearing losses in children. Characteristics, identification, and management. *Pediatric Clinics of North America, 46*, 65–78.

Tilanus, S. C., Van Stenis, D., & Snik, F. M. (1995). Otoacoustic emission measurements in evaluation of the immediate effect of ventilation tube insertion in children. *Annals of Otology, Rhinology, and Laryngology, 104*, 297–300.

van der Drift, J. F. C., Brocaar, M. P., & van Zanten, G. A. (1987). The relation between the pure-tone audiogram and the click auditory brainstem response threshold in cochlear hearing loss. *Audiology, 26*, 1–10.

Ventry, I. M., & Weinstein, B. E. (1982). The Hearing Handicap Inventory for the Elderly: A new tool. *Ear and Hearing, 3*, 128–134.

Ventry, I. M., & Weinstein, B. M., (1983). Identification of elderly people with hearing problems. *Asha, 25*, 37–42.

Weinstein, B. M., & Ventry, I. M. (1983). Audiometric correlates of the Hearing Handicap Inventory for the Elderly. *Journal of Speech and Hearing Disorders, 48*, 379–384.

Yellin, M. W., Jerger, J., & Fifer, R. C. (1989). Norms for disproportionate loss in speech intelligibility. *Ear and Hearing, 10*, 231–234.

The table below, reproduced with permision, shows maximum possible phonetically balanced (PB_{max}) as a function of pure tone average (PTA) at 1000, 2000, and 4000 Hz.

Table 12. Lower boundary of PB_{max} score as a function of PTA_2. For any given value of PTA_2, any score below the tabled value of PB_{max} must be considered disproportionately poor.

PTA_2	PB_{max} (%)	PTA_2	PB_{max} (%)	PTA_2	PB_{max} (%)
0	89	31	57	61	26
1	88	32	56	62	25
2	87	33	55	63	24
3	86	34	54	64	23
4	85	35	53	65	22
5	84	36	52	66	21
6	83	37	51	67	20
7	82	38	50	68	19
8	81	39	49	69	18
9	80	40	48	70	17
10	79	41	47	71	16
11	78	42	46	72	15
12	77	43	45	73	14
13	76	44	44	74	13
14	75	45	43	75	12
15	74	46	42	76	11
16	73	47	41	77	10
17	72	48	40	78	9
18	71	49	39	79	8
19	70	50	38	80	7
20	69	51	37	81	6
21	68	52	36	82	5
22	67	53	35	83	4
23	65	54	34	84	3
24	64	55	32	85	2
25	63	56	31	86	1
26	62	57	30		
27	61	58	29		
28	60	59	28		
29	59	60	27		
30	58				

Yoshinaga-Itano, C., Sedey, A. L., Coulter, D. K., & Mehl, A. L. (1998). Language of early- and later-identified children with hearing loss. Pediatrics, *102*, 1161–1171.

Zhou, G., & Cox, L. C. (2004). Vestibular evoked myogenic potentials: history and overview. *American Journal of Audiology, 13*, 135–143.

Index

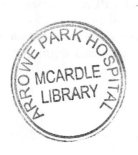